MegaYoga™

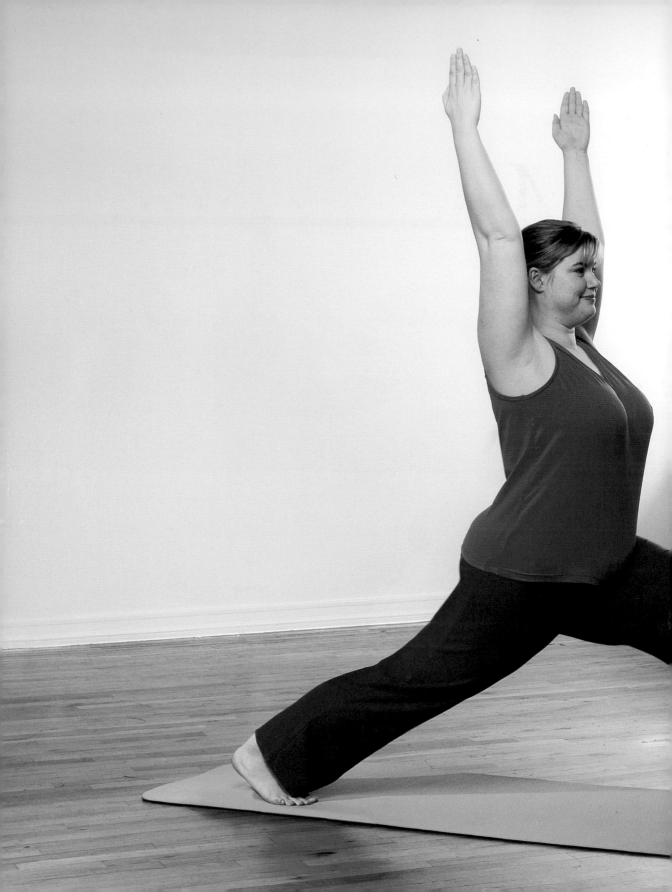

MegaYoga™

Megan Garcia

Photography by
Kellie Walsh

DK Publishing

LONDON, NEW YORK, MELBOURNE,
MUNICH, DELHI

To my students, present and future

Senior Editor Jennifer Williams
Senior Designer Tai Blanche
Managing Art Editor Michelle Baxter
Art Director Dirk Kaufman
DTP Coordinator Kathy Farias
Production Manager Ivor Parker
Executive Managing Editor Sharon Lucas
Publishing Director Carl Raymond

Photography 4 Eyes Photography
Front Cover Photography Nadine Raphael
Hair and Make-up Stylist Tamami Mihara
Consultant Nasim Mawji

First American Edition 2006
06 07 08 09 10 9 8 7 6 5 4 3 2 1

Published in the United States by
DK Publishing
375 Hudson Street
New York, New York 10014

DK books are available at special discounts for bulk purchases for sales
promotions, premiums, fund-raising, or educational use. For details contact
DK Publishing Special Markets, 375 Hudson Street, New York, New York 10014
or SpecialSales@dk.com

Cataloging-in-Publication data is available
from the Library of Congress.
ISBN: 0-7566-1947-5

Color reproduction by Colourscan, Singapore
Printed and bound in China by Sheck Wah Tong Printing Press Ltd.

Discover more at
www.dk.com

CONTENTS

MY JOURNEY

When people see their own image reflected back to them, they see themselves, that they exist, that they belong: Everyone wants to feel worthy of love, just the way they are. My calling has been that of a role model for plus-size women through my work as a yoga instructor promoting a healthy lifestyle, and as a plus-size model celebrating a nontraditional vision of beauty.

Running around the soccer field one afternoon in high school, I thought, "Why am I killing myself to keep up with everyone else?" The girls on my team ran so fast. They didn't have to wear two sports bras or buy their uniform in an extra-large size. They loved winning, leaving their opponents in the dust. I didn't care. I loved breathing, moving, feeling my muscles perform, but the competition and showiness of organized sports left me cold.

I found my perfect match in yoga class in college. From the first moment, I realized that my height and weight were not an issue. Instead, my flexibility lent itself to deep stretching and my loner personality was perfectly in tune with the noncompetitive and meditative elements of yoga practice.

As the semester progressed, I found that I felt great after every class. My body was responding to the postures with gains in flexibility and strength. I met my first challenge during Sun Salute. This postural flow involves stepping back into an upright push-up position and then lowering yourself so that you are hovering several inches above the ground, balancing on your hands and toes. As I was performing the pose, the teacher came over to me and said, "Megan, lift your torso off the ground." It *was* off the ground! But my breasts were resting on the mat, giving the appearance that I was on my stomach. I was so frustrated. I tried to communicate this to my teacher without success.

Next, she taught us Child's pose. Frustrated once again, I found that my stomach was prohibiting me from folding forward. Intuitively, I widened my legs so that my stomach could rest on the mat. In that moment I discovered the first modification for my plus-size body. I knew there was something about yoga that I was called to do, so I kept practicing after graduating from college.

In 1997, I took a trip to Kripalu Center in Lenox, Massachusetts, for a yoga retreat designed just for women. At one point in the workshop the leader passed around paper and boxes of crayons. We were asked to draw images of ourselves. The drawing I did was of a light body with rays of energy shooting out of the core—an image that reflected my feelings whenever I practiced yoga. The other students drew representations of themselves that exaggerated their shapes. During the discussion of the self-portraits, all of the conversation focused on the parts of the body they wanted to change. At that moment, it became clear to me that these women were at war with their bodies. I saw that I was very lucky to feel beautiful and enjoy my body, and that this self-love was a gift. I promised myself that I would never lose this feeling of freedom and energy.

After the retreat I moved to Manhattan to pursue acting and to continue studying yoga, always looking for instruction that would suit my body. After class, other students would approach me and ask about the modifications I had created to make yoga poses work for my body. They looked so relieved that finally someone knew how they felt inside their plus-size bodies. I felt called to teach. In 1999, I went back to Kripalu Center for training. There I received excellent, in-depth instruction on poses, breathing, meditation, and philosophy in the Kripalu tradition.

Megan with husband Rolando Garcia at *Figure* magazine photo shoot

It was my husband who suggested that I try plus-size modeling—a career where my yoga training in concentration and flexibility came to my rescue the first time I had to model winter coats in August! My first national campaign was an ad for a plus-size retailer, and it attracted a lot of attention. I realized that plus-size women like me long for positive role models, women who are confident and out there for all the world to see.

I made a yoga DVD in February of 2005 with the support of one of my modeling clients. It was called *Yoga: Just My Size*™ *with Megan Garcia* and I designed it in the spirit of offering yoga to plus-size women who thought they'd never be be able to practice. I hope MegaYoga™ also inspires them.

Megan Garcia

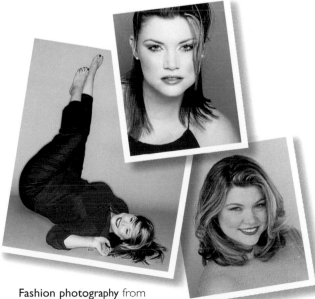

Fashion photography from Megan's modeling portfolio

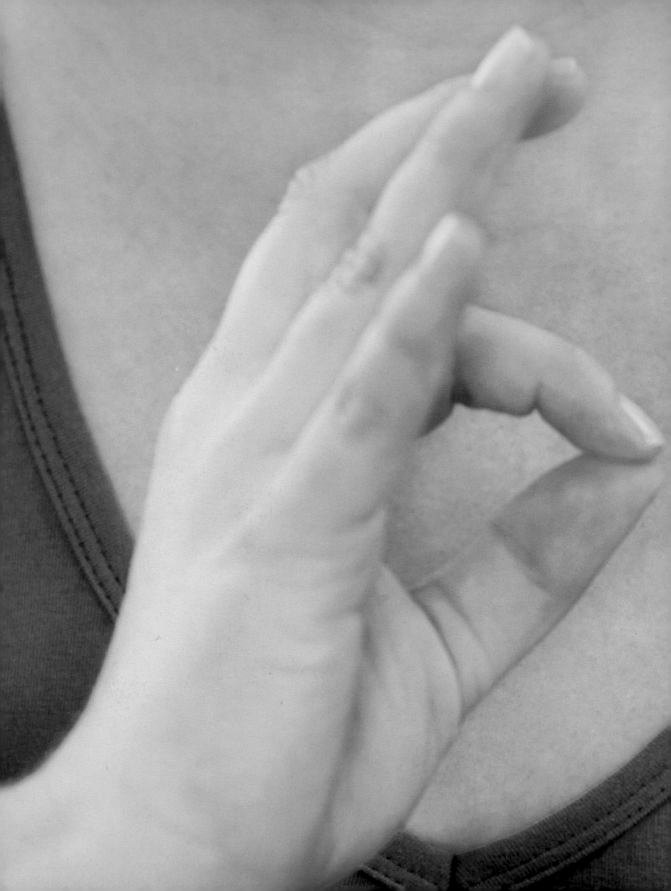

INTRODUCTION TO MEGAYOGA™

MegaYoga™ uses breath, movement, and
meditation to generate strength and sensitivity
in the plus-size body. Regular practice will
provide the practitioner with a greater
knowledge of the workings of her body.
In this introductory section, special skills such
as moving the flesh and binding the breasts are
offered to those of us whose bellies or breasts
make traditional yoga postures uncomfortable
or impossible. These modifications, including
the use of props, and understanding the basics
of yogic breathing and proper alignment,
make the work accessible to all women.

WHAT IS MEGAYOGA™?

MegaYoga™ is the practice of hatha (movement) yoga, modified for plus-size women. It includes unique adaptations, such as moving the flesh and breast binding, and is designed to strengthen and sensitize the practitioner, while bringing her home to her body: Coming face to face with all the secrets and scars, both inner and outer, that have become imprinted on the flesh can be frightening. MegaYoga™ gives the plus-size woman the tools to befriend her body, to gain greater self-confidence, and to win a new sense of freedom, as she moves forward through her life.

EMPOWERMENT

The poses in every chapter of MegaYoga™ are designed to have an uplifting and empowering effect on the practitioner. Although MegaYoga™ programs are intended for beginners, I have included some ambitious balancing poses such as Warrior 1 (see p68–69), Half Moon (see p82–83) and Handstand (see p100–101) to challenge and build up the internal and muscular strength of the plus-size practitioner. Unlike many yoga and fitness programs, weight loss is not the goal of MegaYoga™—although it may be the result for some. Rather, it is to empower the practitioner to become more aware of the needs and inner workings of her body. I remember my first body revelations— the moment when I was able to feel my ribs move in Dirgha breathing (see pp26–27) and the feeling of exultation the first time I was able to hold myself in Handstand (see p100–101) for more than a few breaths.

SELF-CONFIDENCE

Plus-size women face many challenges on a daily basis simply because of our size. Many of us consequently shut down and regard our bodies as a source of frustration and embarrassment. Some of us experience social ostracism for not conforming to the standards of what is considered beautiful in the prevailing culture. Many of us have to struggle to find nice clothing that fits, to fit into seats on airplanes and public transportation, to feel that we belong in a fitness class full of smaller bodies. These challenges are surmountable when we know we can master a tricky yoga pose: One small victory over doubt and muscle fatigue can snowball into standing taller, prouder, and being unafraid to be seen. It takes hard work to challenge yourself through a physical discipline like yoga, but the rewards are great.

SENSITIVITY

In addition to empowerment and self-confidence, MegaYoga™ teaches students about sensitivity. This work occurs in the breathing methods practiced in MegaYoga™ (see Breathing pp26–29). Breathing slowly and deeply enables you to focus on everything your body is feeling. If you are blessed with all your senses, you will have endless opportunities to savor a delicate perfume, bask in the warmth of the sun, taste freshly baked bread, enjoy a piano sonata, see the face of your beloved. In MegaYoga™ we fine-tune the sense of touch. You will massage your own feet, stretch, and luxuriate in heating and cooling your body. You will find, as you work, that your breath and the energy that lies dormant in your body is quite sensual. It is pleasurable to flirt with elevating this energy. The first layer of sweat that breaks out as you warm up wakes you up. As your senses awaken you will become aware of all the thoughts and sensations that are suppressed when your breathing is shallow, and you will naturally commit to breathing deeper.

MAKING ADJUSTMENTS

Although MegaYoga™ is firmly planted in the tradition of hatha yoga (yoga that involves movement), the element that makes it completely unique is the practitioner—plus-size women—and the method, which fine-tunes traditional yoga postures to suit the special needs of larger bodies. For example, we need props to help us balance and reach; we need to know which poses are contraindicated by our weight; we need to physically move and readjust our flesh in specific ways to glean the most benefit from our practice; and we must be particularly aware of safe alignment, so that our joints are not overstressed. These special considerations are addressed at length in Yoga Props (pp2l–2l), Getting Started (pp24–25), Moving the Flesh (pp22–23), General Alignment (ppl6–l7) and Guidelines for Practice (ppl8–l9).

COMING HOME TO YOUR BODY

Like all people, we are hungry for love. I learn so much from my students—they are drawn to yoga for the same reason that I and all students are drawn to it—connection with ourselves and with the divine. This union occurs through the breath.

When my students begin to practice I remind them over and over again to be conscious of their breath—and its intimate connection with our emotions. I encourage them to breathe through painful feelings, to stay with their breath. I believe that emotions that are not consciously processed are stored in the body. I experienced this as a college student when my grandmother died. I had to fly home right away for the funeral and then rush back to school for exams. When I woke up in my dorm room my neck had frozen completely. I couldn't turn my head more than an inch without great pain. I had tried my best not to cry at my grandmother's funeral because I was responsible for reading her eulogy. It's no coincidence that all the held breath and choked-back tears resulted in a paralyzing muscle spasm. Without breath we clench up. Maybe you've had a similar experience—like a stomachache after an argument or a sore throat before an important speech. Breath work in MegaYoga™ teaches us how to breathe through our emotions so that we don't panic when we are faced with painful feelings.

ACCEPTANCE

If you can learn how to be in a pose without judging how you are doing compared to other students, you will be practicing MegaYoga™—Enjoy the practice without harsh self-judgments and use your breath to stay focused and observe what is happening to you on the basic level of sensations. It will not be easy. But if you can begin to have moments of concentration you will most surely gain greater freedom in your body.

I hope you will avoid the shadowy side of body awakening, which is slavishly fixated on the outer form we take. Rather, use your practice to learn more about yourself, and then take that knowledge and change whatever doesn't work for you. As you travel this path, always remember to treat yourself with compassion.

I encourage you to keep growing and thriving in your practice. Remember that you are not traveling on the path of yoga alone.

HEALTH BENEFITS

The poses and breathing techniques in MegaYoga™ work together to affect your body, down to a cellular level. Through the transformative power of regular practice you will gain greater lung capacity, improved balance and strength, and better sleep and digestion. The challenge for you will be to remain open to any hindrances you may face—whether it's a tight set of hamstrings or the fear of turning upside down. Be kind to yourself when you struggle and celebrate the benefits as they come along.

PHYSICAL STRENGTH

In Warm-ups (see pp30–63) and Standing Poses (see pp64–91), you will strengthen your muscles and improve your balance. These dual attributes are especially important for plus-size practitioners because our weight puts pressure on our joints, which can lead to stiffness, pain, and possibily for some, arthritis. Strong muscles help support and stabilize our joints so that we can move without pain. Without strong abdominal muscles and buttocks, the added weight from generous bellies can cause the pelvis to tip forward, increasing the curvature in the lower back, and leading to lower back pain or weakness. Many students in my classes have this postural tendency as well as difficulty getting up and down from the floor without undue effort or pain. Mindful Standing (see pp60–63) addresses getting up and down from the floor using leg strength. In the Warm-ups (see pp30–63), Table Balance (see p52) helps develop abdominal strength. All of the lunging and squatting postures in Standing Poses (see p64–91) work on developing the strength of the buttocks.

BALANCE

Standing Poses (see pp64–91) such as Half Moon (see pp 82–83) and inversions such as Handstand (see pp 100–101) develop your stabilizer muscles that help you sense when you are off balance. I used to stand and wait for the subway or bus with one hip cocked and all my weight on my right leg. Over time, standing this

way misaligns your hips so that it feels "correct." After I made the connection between my daily postural habits and the symptoms of poor alignment that began to show up on my yoga mat, I made a determined effort to stand in a balanced fashion.

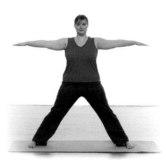

Regular movement cleanses our organs and helps our bodies fight infection.

GRACE

In each step of every yoga pose in this book you will see instructions on how to breathe. Consciously inhaling or exhaling with a movement develops the skill of moving gracefully. Try this: Without breathing, bring your arms up off the page and lift them above your head, like a dancer. Really get into it. Now stop and breathe deeply. Inhale as you lift your arms, exhale as you lower them. Doesn't the motion seem almost effortless?

INNER CLEANSING

Cleansing Poses (see pp108–123) such as Wind Reliever (see pp120–121) and Fish (see p110) work on your internal organs, helping metabolic processes, digestion, and elimination. Twisting poses flush the inner organs with a fresh supply of oxygenated blood when you release the pose. Seated and reclining twists irrigate the kidneys, organs that process waste in the body, while other cleansers such as Happy Baby (see pp114–115) help eliminate excess gas so that you can digest the food you eat with more comfort. Regular movement will help keep your body processing wastes, draining fluids from swollen tissues, and digesting and fighting off infections.

LOWER BLOOD PRESSURE

When I went in for a check-up recently, my doctor told me she was going to take a second blood pressure reading after my general exam. When I asked her why, she told me that most people are anxious when they arrive at the doctor's office, and the first reading is generally a bit elevated. After the patient has had a chance to relax and breathe more deeply, the second blood pressure reading is lower. Imagine the wonderful effects of an entire hour of yoga practice on your blood pressure and your heart. When you soothe yourself with deep Dirgha breathing (see pp26–27), your entire system benefits during—and after— yoga practice.

Standing poses build strength, balance, and body confidence. With regular practice, you will enjoy many changes as you get to know your body better.

TOOLS FOR LIVING

Practicing yoga is more than poses and breathing. Around the third century AD the yogic sage Patanjali codified the practice of yoga in his Yoga Sutras (Threads) and constructed an ethical code of Do's and Dont's on topics such as self-love, truthfulness, contentment, compassion, and discipline. Most major religions have ethical codes, such as the Ten Commandments in Chritianity, and while yoga is not a religion, it nevertheless suggests guidelines for ethical living that are as relevant today as they were in Patanjali's time.

DISCIPLINE

Your body is constantly sending you signals for its preservation. Through the practice of yoga you learn to tune in to them. For example, I have a student who always held her breath on the exhale in Dirgha breathing (see p26–27). There was no physical reason for this. Eventually she realized that the grief she carried over the death of a loved one made it frightening for her to let go of her breath—she was afraid she would cry. But when she created a warm and safe container for her breath by gently and slowly warming up her body she was able to let herself exhale and cry so that she didn't have to keep suppressing her feelings. This revelation changed her life for the better. You will receive many gifts from your body if you listen closely. Yoga helps translate aches and fears into a story.

What's the catch? You will only be able to hear what your body is saying if you practice long enough and often enough. Without committing yourself, you won't stick with the program when you start sweating or aching or become bored. It is only by pushing yourself a bit that you can elevate your heart rate or strengthen weak muscles. It is only by trying a scary pose—an inversion perhaps—that you will gain the confidence to take on more challenges. Commit to practicing the 30-Minute Program (see p140–143) for one week. Notice what happens when you commit to regular practice.

SELF-LOVE

Yoga gives me dignity. I've noticed that plus-size women in the subway here in New York seem ashamed when they sit down and spill over onto the seat next to them. They shrink into themselves and try to become invisible. I've also noticed lots of men—big and small—who sprawl their legs and take up two seats without shame. In MegaYoga™ we proudly take up space. It begins with allowing our bellies to inflate fully as we breathe as deeply as we can (see Breathing, p26–29). Then in the standing poses (see pp64–91) we purposely spread ourselves out to take up space for a good stretch. After a lifetime of trying not to impose, take up two seats, or get noticed, it can be liberating to allow your body to express itself. Don't shrink away from yourself. Stand tall.

TRUTHFULNESS

My body and maybe yours doesn't look like the bodies of lots of yoga practitioners. If I pretend that I don't have ample breasts or a belly, I will be uncomfortable in some yoga postures—for example, compressing my breasts in a low lunge. Acknowledging the truth about my body shape lets me make modifications for my comfort and safety. By making an honest account of my level of fitness I am able to avoid moves that I am not ready to practice yet and thereby avoid potential injury.

COMPASSION

After being truthful about my body I immediately face the challenge of the judging mind that says "Why are you so different? Your breasts are too big, etc." This sort of negative self-talk is not helpful for our development as loving beings. We wouldn't talk that way to our child, to our loved ones. When you are adjusting your body (see Moving the Flesh, p22–23) in order to accommodate your body to various poses in MegaYoga™, I ask that you do so without making negative comments about your flesh, the size of your body, etc. Simply be in the moment and move what you need to move. Be disciplined about practicing positive self-talk. You can only cultivate peace and contentment if you speak to yourself from a place of compassion.

CONTENTMENT

In Getting Started (pp24–25) I talk about some of the things you need to begin practicing yoga—but you may need less than you think. So many of us get caught up in acquiring things as an excuse not to get started. When I went to yoga teacher training, I found that during meditation I was making a mental list of everything I wanted to buy when I got home—inspirational CDs, books, cool-looking yoga gear, etc., etc. I wasn't really present in the meditation at all! When you are caught up in desiring and coveting things, you are off in a fantasy land, instead of being present in your life. When this happens, don't beat yourself up—just take a deep breath and concentrate on what you are doing right now. Be content to live in the moment.

Yoga is an ancient discipline that continues to resonate in our time. As long as you seek better health and inner peace yoga will be helpful.

GENERAL ALIGNMENT

It may be challenging to get a good sense of your own skeletal structure, especially if you're a plus-size practitioner—we have a tricky time palpating through layers of flesh to find the bony landmarks of our anatomy. Spend some time studying the image of the female pelvis, below, to get a better sense of the underlying structure of your skeleton. Also examine the points of balance on your feet (see p17). The annotations of Mountain pose, to the right, also point out important elements of standing with good posture.

ALIGNMENT FOR WOMEN

I received invaluable instruction on safe alignment for women from yoga and anatomy expert, Adrienne Jamiel, RYT. She explains that hatha yoga, the yoga of movement, was created in India by Brahman men. The men mastered good alignment in standing poses based on the shape of their skeletons. When women began to practice yoga, they were taught the same alignment technique because it was the only one. However, if you take a look at the anatomical drawings to the left, you will see the difference between male and female pelvic structure. Women have a wider pelvis so that we can deliver babies vaginally, through the birth canal. Therefore, we have more of a separation between our legs. In some yoga classes students are told to align their feet with the inside edges touching. Try doing this right now. Put the book down and see how it feels to stand in this fashion. When I do this I feel wobbly and off balance. Now align your feet so that they are under your hips, bone stacking on top of bone. Begin by hopping up and down in place. Jump lightly so that your feet leave the ground for just a second. Don't overanalyze it. Just hop. Now land. Notice where your feet are. Do you feel stable? Try this again and again noticing that every time you land with your feet under you—not touching. Try landing with your feet together. Very hard, right? Your hips are womanly and wide and your stance needs to reflect that for your comfort. Thank you, Adrienne, for this intuitive and enlightening teaching.

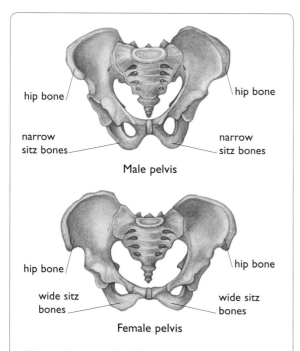

hip bone / hip bone

narrow sitz bones / narrow sitz bones

Male pelvis

hip bone / hip bone

wide sitz bones / wide sitz bones

Female pelvis

Your pelvis is much wider than a man's, and so are your sitz bones. The next time you're sitting down, reach under your buttocks and feel where your sitz bones are—they are the bones you sit on.

keep shoulders relaxed back and down

lift chest

Whenever you practice Mountain (see pp66–67), the first standing pose, always begin by hopping to find the hip width that is true for your pelvis. When you take a yoga class in your community, don't allow yourself to feel pressured to align your feet in any way that does not work for your body. Explain the hopping method to your teacher, if you need to.

When you are standing in Mountain pose, keep your chest lifted and shoulders back. Squeeze your thigh and buttock muscles to support your back.
Your feet should be parallel, your knees soft. Press up through the crown of your head and down into the soles of your feet.

POINTS OF BALANCE

The feet are the foundation of every Standing pose (see p64–91). Proper weight distribution will improve your balance and help you derive maximum benefit from the poses. Always begin every standing pose by checking the placement of your feet. Note that the three points of the foot shown below support the arches on the sole.

1) The ball of the big toe

2) The ball of the little toe

3) The heel

You may notice that the outside or inside edge of your shoe wears down on one side more than the other—the result of placing more or less pressure on either Point 1 or Point 2. Work in your yoga practice to put even pressure on all three points when you stand. You'll notice that the three points have the same effect as a tripod to keep you upright and balanced.

squeeze thigh muscles and buttocks to support the spine

keep knees soft, never locked

keep feet parallel, hip-width apart for maximum stability

Mountain pose

GUIDELINES FOR PRACTICE

Now that you are familiar with the anatomy of your pelvis, you can use this information to achieve good seated posture as well as learn how to center yourself before you begin your yoga practice. Sitting erect, using your skeleton to balance in natural alignment, means that your muscles don't have to work so hard to keep you upright, and you can stay seated or standing in a pose longer, without undue fatigue or strain. Achieving active standing poses while preserving joint stability is another essential component of practicing yoga safely and enjoyably.

FINDING YOUR BONES FOR SEATED POSTURES

Now that you are familiar with the shape of a woman's pelvis, think about what happens to yours when you sit down on your bottom. If you are sitting tall, without strain, you are balancing on the base of your pelvis, on the sitz bones, which are covered with a layer of muscle and fat. To feel where they are, and to check your alignment, sit on a hard chair or the bare floor. Reach behind you and pull back the flesh of your buttocks until you can feel the two bones at the base of your

pelvis. Now rock forward onto the head of the bones, tipping the top of your pelvis forward, toward your feet. Next, rock through the center, backward onto the back of the sitz bones, tipping the top of your pelvis toward the wall behind you. How does your lower back feel? I notice a strain in mine, as my spine grips to compensate for losing balance and falling backward. Bring your pelvis to

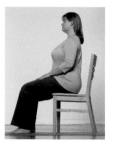

Try to sit tall, without leaning on the backrest, if you are more comfortable sitting in a chair.

center by rolling onto the center of your sitz bones at all times. In this alignment your spine can grow tall without bending forward or backward. Also, you will be prepared for centering—15 to 20 minutes of essential quiet time before you begin your yoga practice.

Centering (see photo, left) is used to focus the mind and calm the heart. Find a quiet place to concentrate on deep breathing and introspection before you begin your practice with Warm-Ups (see p30-63). Many yoga classes begin with a chant, but if you feel more comfortable listening and breathing deeply, that is perfectly fine.

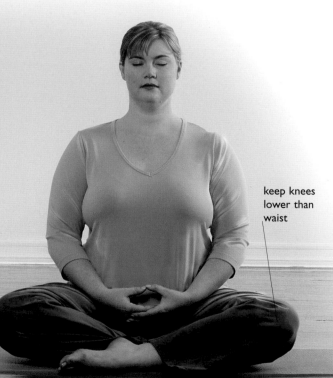

keep knees
lower than
waist

In a seated, centered posture, my pelvis is level—rolled neither forward nor backward. This takes strain off my spine and allows me to sit longer in comfort.

JOINT SAFETY

In yoga postures, where a joint will bear weight for a period of time—for example, a lunge in Mindful Standing (see pp60–63), Warrior 1 and Warrior 2 (see pp68–71), and Awkward pose (see pp90–91)—you must stabilize it so it does not move, and make sure not to bend it past the normal range of motion.

STABILITY

The ability to engage (squeeze) the muscles of your legs is a crucial skill in yoga. Sit down on the floor and pull up your pants leg so that you can see and feel your thigh muscles. Now reach down and touch your kneecap. Slide it up and down vertically. Feel how it moves. Now squeeze the muscles of your thigh as hard as you can. Try to move the kneecap while maintaining the squeeze. Can't do it? That's stability. In Standing Poses (see pp64–91) I will ask you to engage the muscles of the thighs as you enter into postures where your legs bear weight. Remember this action and feeling.

NORMAL RANGE OF MOTION

When you lunge, make sure that the knee of your bent leg does not go past a 90° angle in order to avoid straining the joint. A quick test is to take a lunge and glance down to see if you can see the top of your forward foot and all of your toes.

The second part of the safety check is to be sure that the joint is aligned. Notice when you lunge whether your knee points toward the outside or the inside edge of your foot. It should track directly over the middle toes. As you go into Tree pose (see pp76–77), place your foot anywhere on your leg except at the side of the knee. The kneecaps slide up and down as you walk. Be mindful not to put any torque on the kneecap so that it doesn't move from side to side.

keep ears aligned over shoulders to prevent head from jutting forward

keep shoulder blades moving back and down to keep spine long and posture tall

keep hipbones facing forward to prevent twisting back

squeeze thigh muscles to keep hip from dropping and moving pelvis out of alignment

knee should be over center of foot at a 90° angle or less

make sure you can see all of your toes when you look down

YOGA PROPS

Props enable us to enter into—and stay longer in—poses that would otherwise be too difficult to achieve without support, particularly those that involve lunges and inversions. References to specialized props, and how to use them, appear throughout the book in Modifying the Pose and Intensifying the Pose boxes.

WALLS AND CHAIRS

Props help us stay upright in balancing poses. For example, we lean against a wall when we learn Tree Pose (see pp76–77) or against a chair in Forward Fold Rest (see p84) and Down Dog (see pp98–99).

YOGA STRAPS

Props help us reach further. For example, I like to use a yoga strap to stretch my hamstrings in Reclining Leg Stretch (see pp116–117) while keeping my shoulders relaxed on the floor. We also use a yoga strap in Shoulder Opener (see p85) to prepare ourselves for the big stretch in Stargazer (seee pp86–87). Yoga straps are also very useful in binding the breasts, a technique I explain in Moving the Flesh (see pp22–23).

BOLSTERS AND BLOCKS

Props support our bodies so that we can achieve and stay in postures without strain. A good example is putting a bolster or a cushion under one buttock in Pigeon (see p128–129) or under both buttocks in various seated postures to keep the pelvis upright and the spine long and tall. I use a yoga block or a chair to reach the floor in standing poses such as Triangle (see p78–79) or Half Moon (see p82–83). Instructions on how to use yoga props are usually illustrated in the packaging that comes with them. Props are also quite easy to improvise from things you already have at home, so don't worry about spending a lot of money on them.

Straps

Bolster

Yoga mat

Blocks

Some of the props used in MegaYoga™ are blocks, chairs, yoga mats, bolsters, yoga straps or ties—and even the walls of your home.

STICKY YOGA MATS

A yoga prop that is now omnipresent in the media, and associated with the way yoga is practiced in America, is the sticky yoga mat, so called because the materials used in manufacturing the mats provide extra traction. We use sticky mats in this book to highlight the positioning of the feet and body, and because they provide a bit of padding on a hard floor. My students use them in my yoga classes because I rent space and cannot always be sure that the wood floors are pristine. For some of my plus-size students with sensitive knees, the padding that regular-width sticky mats provide is not enough to cushion their hands and knees. For warm-up poses, I recommend that they use an extra-thick sticky mat plus a blanket folded into thirds. Place the blanket horizontally across the mat to form a cross. Rest your knees on the folded blanket to provide maximum cushioning for the entire kneeling section.

WHEN TO UNSTICK YOURSELF

As you progress you will be ready to challenge your stabilizer muscles (the muscles that hold your joints in place). I believe that sticky mats are not a helpful tool in the long term (after a steady year of practice) because the stickiness does the work your stabilizer muscles should do—keeping your feet from sliding apart. I practice yoga at home on an oriental rug without a mat. The rug is nice and thick for the sake of my knees so I don't have to sacrifice padding. One of my teachers at Kripalu Center practiced yoga before there were sticky mats. He would practice in the chapel at Kripalu, which has wall-to-wall carpeting. Sometimes in the winter he would even wear wool socks during his practice because he was cold. He found that his inner and outer thighs became very strong as he did his standing postures since they worked to prevent his feet from sliding. I'm not up to wearing socks on the carpet, and I can't recommend what I don't do. But I have found that practicing without the sticky surface gives me a big inner-thigh challenge.

LOOK INWARD

I do not recommend using a mirror for plus-size practitioners: The temptation to judge the body is too great. I work very hard to simply feel sensations in my body when I struggle and sweat in a pose. If I were to look in a mirror, ostensibly for the purpose of checking alignment, I would be tempted to judge the way I look in the pose. (Watch students in a yoga class—they all check each other out.) Your body will not look like mine when you do the poses in this book—it will look like your body! Be careful not to judge yourself unfairly when you use props, especially in yoga class, where there's a tendency to be competitive. Do you feel less "competent" or less "advanced" than people who don't use props? Do you feel like you're no good at a pose because you use a chair, a strap, or a cushion? If you do, throw that judgment right out the window, and remember that a prop is just a prop. As long as you can get into a pose, stay in it, and enjoy it, it doesn't matter how you got there!

PROPS AT HOME AND IN CLASS

You can start practicing yoga at home as soon as you like—no special props are required. Everything you need is readily available: You have a wall, a door, and chairs for support in balancing and inverted poses. A cushion from your couch works just as well as a yoga bolster, and you can use a blanket from your bed instead of a yoga mat. A men's necktie or a bathrobe belt makes an excellent yoga strap and you can use two phone books or dictionaries instead of yoga blocks.

If you take a yoga class in your community, I recommend that you come in early to set up your props. If you would like to use a wall or chairs, you should inform the teacher ahead of time and set yourself up before class begins. Don't scramble mid-practice to go get a blanket or a pillow. This disturbs your fellow practitioners. I recommend that you also wait until the teacher has concluded the class before folding up your mat, straps, or any other prop.

MOVING THE FLESH

For our comfort, we learn to "move the flesh" in MegaYoga™ warm-ups and poses. This concept is a radical departure from most exercise regimens, where ample flesh is deemed excessive, and the primary motivation is to work it off. In my opinion, this focus is incompatible with the true spirit of yoga, in which we practice ahimsa and satya—nonviolence and truth. The idea is to practice without causing the body or the mind pain, pain that surely is felt when your belly is perceived as "in your way." The virtue of truth is important for a practitioner, who must realize that all of her flesh is her own: This belly, these thighs are all you. See them and feel them as you practice without judgment.

MOVING PRINCIPLES

This concept is one of the keys to adapting classic yoga postures to our bodies. When I first practiced forward bends, my hips were open enough to allow me to bend forward, but my belly prevented me from completing the pose. To my flat-stomached friends, I liken this phenomenon to having a big feather pillow tied to your torso. I learned that the layers of fat in the belly are soft enough to move easily: When I take hold of my belly and smooth it in and up I can bend forward, freeing the hip joint. Always move your flesh *away* from the joint that will be moving. Touch yourself gently and patiently as you move your flesh. You have all the time in the world. Remember to breathe.

lift the flesh up with your fingertips

In Eagle Pose (see pp88–89) I need to move my inner thigh flesh out to the side in order to press my legs together. Most plus-size women can really relate to this.

ADJUSTMENTS

All of us have different bodies. You will have to use your own body awareness to figure out if your movements are impeded by inflexibility or by the position of your flesh. The clue to recognizing the difference between the two is breath. I've found that I can still breathe easily when I'm stopped by a tight muscle, but I start to feel suffocated when I'm bending into and compressing flesh, especially

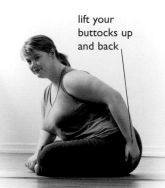

lift your buttocks up and back

Any seated posture begins with finding your sitz bones (see p16). No matter what your size, make a point of finding your pelvic alignment whenever you sit down.

in my belly. Another time to move the flesh is if you are going into a movement but have to strain around your flesh to complete the pose. For example, in Seated Twist (see p36) some students find that when they twist, their belly stops rotating because it hits their thigh. At this point if they want to continue to twist they must move their belly up and in so that they do not transfer the main thrust of the twist into their upper back and neck. Another example is the lunge. Students with large breasts find that when they take a kneeling lunge the breast on the side of the forward leg is crushed by that leg (I speak from personal experience here). The student must slide her breast to the inside of the bent leg when she lunges so as not to contort the knee of the bent leg away from the breast in an effort to relieve the pressure.

In the blue box (right) there are two examples of body shapes of yoga practitioners. These shapes are neither good nor bad; one is not sexier than the other. Rather, the shapes describe where we carry our body weight. Learning your own shape will help you make modifications for your comfort as you practice yoga. You may not have either shape. That's okay. Use any modifications that help you.

TWO COMMON BODY TYPES

Apple students have larger torsos than hourglass students. They are challenged by any pose that compresses their abdomen. If you carry your weight in your belly, you will need to move the flesh in seated twists and forward bends.

Hourglass students have larger busts and hips than apple students. I am an hourglass. We are challenged by upside down poses and need to bind our breasts for these. Balancing poses can be a challenge as well, so we use chairs or a wall for support.

BINDING THE BREASTS

I have found an unusual use for the yoga strap. I use it to bind my breasts so that when I bend forward they do not fall into my face and impede my breathing. Not all of you will need this modification, but if you have large breasts like me you will find the strap useful in forward-bending poses such as Down Dog (see pp98–99) and Dolphin (see pp102–103), and in upside down poses such as Bridge (see pp112–113) and Half Shoulder Stand (see pp106–107), where the breasts fall back, covering the neck and pressing on the chin. As always, you are your own best teacher. In this book I am shown without the strap so that women of all shapes can relate to the poses. Try the poses with the strap and without and see which version you prefer. To use the strap, click the ends into place, forming a big loop. Slip the loop over your head and shoulders and under your armpits. Pull on the end of the strap, as shown in the photo (right) to tighten the loop, compressing your breasts. Once you have applied it, make sure it does not slip when you lift your arms. The strap should be very snug when applied properly.

In any of the upside down poses, binding the breasts flattens your breasts so that your nose and mouth are not covered and you can breathe easily.

make sure the strap fits snugly, even when you lift your arms up

GETTING STARTED

I'm good at starting new projects. The trick for me is staying the course. Perhaps this is true for you, too. I find that making it a goal to practice every day motivates me to get started. On this page you'll find helpful tips on how to set up your space at home for practice, what to wear, and when to practice. How To Use This Book (see opposite page) gives you information about how MegaYoga™ poses should be practiced and what you can learn from the various boxes that accompany each of the poses.

THE PERFECT YOGA SPACE

Fantasy: You find an extra room in your home to dedicate to yoga and contemplation. You have a gleaming wood floor that is pristine. You set up an altar with incense and exotic fresh flowers. You play a CD of temple bells as you wrap yourself in your Pashmina shawl spun from the hairs of free-range Buddhist mountain goats.

Reality: You push aside the dirty laundry to clear a little section on the bedroom floor that is just big enough for you to almost lie down. Then you notice, during a forward bend, that the dust bunnies are breeding under your bed. You feel guilty and compelled to vacuum the floor because it is annoying you.

WHERE & HOW TO PRACTICE

OK, most days my practice is more reality than fantasy. Here in New York, in even the most luxurious yoga studios, you can still hear the traffic. There is no place that is perfectly clean, perfectly serene. As a consequence, I've learned the most important skill to master as a yoga practitioner: how to concentrate. I choose to concentrate all my attention on the sensations of my body and just let the chaos be. If you are practicing at home, there will be many distractions. Aside from turning off things that beep or ring (e.g., alarm clocks, cell phones, etc.) you will have to let the chaos go. Your family or roommate will try to get your attention, the dust bunnies will call to you, you will remember important ideas you just have

to jot down as you are practicing. Just let them be. Don't try to block out the thoughts or distractions. You will get to them just as soon as you are done.

WHAT TO WEAR

You don't need to buy anything special to wear to practice yoga—put on a pair of bottoms that have a waistband that let you breathe deeply. No tight waists! At home, when nobody's watching, I wear pajama bottoms that have a tie. As for tops, you don't want to struggle with a shirt billowing into your face when you turn upside down. Tuck your top into the waistband of your pants for inverted postures. I recommend wearing a softcup bra. Underwires restrict your breathing in breath work. Practice barefoot so that you can see the action of your feet, especially in all standing poses, so that you can sense the three points of balance (see p17).

WHEN TO PRACTICE

The best time to practice is in the morning. All of the fluids in your body pool as you lie prone overnight, but if you begin your day with gentle yoga movements you will stimulate the lymph and circulatory systems so that you feel less puffy and stiff throughout the day. If the morning is not an option for you, you can practice at night. Evening practice will prepare your body for sleep with deep breathing and conscious relaxation.

Do not eat before yoga practice. One forward bend with a full stomach will teach you this lesson quickly. I feel best when I practice about 2–3 hours after a meal.

HOW TO USE THIS BOOK

MegaYoga™ is meant to flow as a complete program, starting with Warm-ups (see pp30–63) and continuing through Standing Poses (see pp64–91), Wall Poses and Inversions (see pp92–107), Cleansing Poses (see pp108–123), and Quiet Poses (see pp124–137). The poses in each of the chapters should be practiced sequentially in order to give you the maximum benefit of each pose. Always begin with Warm-ups until you are sweating lightly. You will then be ready to progress to the postures that follow: Standing Poses, Wall Poses and Inversions, Cleansing Poses, etc. If you are a beginner who would like to ease into practice, or if you have only a limited amount of time to practice, choose the 30-Minute Program (see pp140–143). As you learn all the Warm-ups, combine them, as you wish, with poses in the 60-Minute Program (see pp144–147) and 90-Minute Program (see pp148–152). Always finish with Corpse Pose (seee pp134–135) and Meditation (see pp136–137) to seal the effects of your practice.

Throughout MegaYoga™ there are special boxes that offer different kinds of information about each pose:

• Mega Tip: Offers helpful ways to approach the pose

• Modifying the Pose: Suggests how to do the pose in the most gentle way, sometimes using a prop such as a chair or a cushion

• Intensifying the Pose: Shows advanced students how to make the pose more challenging

• Caution: Gives important medical warnings about the pose. For example, if you have high blood pressure, you should avoid poses that place your head below the level of your heart. Instead, practice gentler modifications that enable you to keep your head level with your heart.

The most important caution I can offer is: Let your body be your teacher. If you feel a stab inside your knee, for example, do not proceed. Back off and rest. You should feel no sensations inside a joint. If you feel sore a day after practice, take a warm bath with Epsom salts and drink lots of water.

You already have everything you need to start practicing MegaYoga™. You've set an intention to strengthen your body and soothe your spirit. That is enough.

BREATHING

In MegaYoga™, we practice three forms of breathing. Dirgha breathing (please see below) helps you breathe deeply at all times—in life as well as on the yoga mat. It is used in all MegaYoga™ postures, except for Standing Poses (see pp64–91), where powerful Ujjayi breathing (see p28) is used to aid concentration. Alternate Nostril Breathing (see pp28–29) is deeply soothing and is used only for Meditation (see pp136–137).

PRANAYAMA

Pranayama is a Sanksrit word that means breath mastery: Prana means energy or breath and ayama means mastery. The practice of breath mastery enables you to take in more oxygen. More oxygen helps you feel energized and think more clearly. Breathing deeply improves digestion and elimination, and slows the heart so that it doesn't have to work so hard. Breathing enables you to experience your feelings more intensely. Conversely, we sometimes hold our breath to insulate ourselves from powerful feelings—witness people about to see a car crash in a movie or a toddler about to get a shot. In fact, the expression "waiting with baited breath" implies anxiety and tension. Take a deep breath right now and let out a sigh: "Ahhhhh." How do you feel? Did you yawn spontaneously? Did your shoulders melt down a little bit?

YOUR BREATHING ANATOMY

It is important to understand the basic anatomy of your lungs before your begin Dirgha breathing. Your lungs reside in the chest cavity above your abdominal organs. Separating the two cavities is a flexible muscle called the diaphragm, which is shaped like a dome. When you inhale, the diaphragm moves down to make room for your lungs to inflate. When the diaphragm moves down it presses on the abdominal organs and this is why you see your belly get bigger when you inhale deeply. When you exhale, the diaphragm moves up, as the lungs deflate, and the air rushes out.

PREPARATION

Blow your nose before you begin. If your throat feels dry, drink some lukewarm water to keep it moist. If you are taking antihistamines, it is especially important to drink lots of water before and during practice to keep yourself hydrated. Don't wear strong perfume or burn incense or candles that are heavily scented because it can stuff up your nose. I owe my understanding of Dirgha breathing technique (see below) to the staff at Kripalu Center, and especially to my instructors Yoganand Michael Carroll and Tarika Diana Damelio.

DIRGHA BREATHING

Dirgha breathing utilizes the entire capacity of your lungs and teaches you how to take in the maximum amount of breath. For a perfect example of this natural, complete breath, watch the belly movement of a sleeping baby. We lose the ease of this elemental breathing as physical and mental tensions accumulate with age, but you can reclaim it with Dirgha breathing each time you practice yoga.

Sit comfortably with your pelvis level and your spine long. You may wish to sit on a cushion to elevate your hips or use a chair. Let out a few sighs and maybe a yawn, then close your lips. Breathing in and out through your nose, place your hands on your belly. We breathe through the nose in yoga because it contains little hairs that filter out dust in the air. Take a moment to review the photos of Step 1–Step 3 of Dirgha breathing (see photos, opposite page) before you begin:

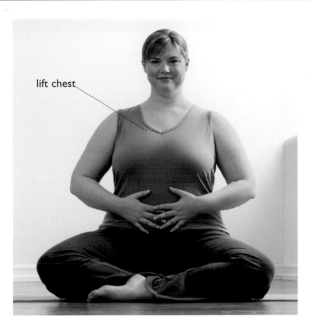

lift chest

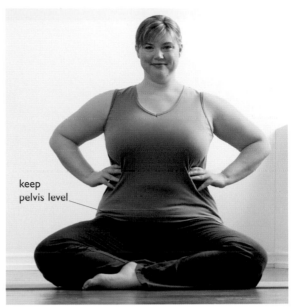

keep
pelvis level

1 Press your hands on your belly. As you inhale, feel your belly inflate like a balloon. Exhale through your nose, and press your belly in toward your spine, letting all the air rush out past your nostrils.

2 Move your hands up to your ribs. Feel how you breathe side to side, not just front to back. Feel your ribs swing in and then out again like an accordion when you inhale and then exhale.

keep shoulders
back and down

3 The third part of Dirgha breathing is in the upper chest. This is where most of us breathe all the time. Place your hands on your chest, below your collarbone. You are touching the large bone of the breastbone. Inhale and feel it lift lightly into your hands. Exhale and feel it fall. Now repeat all the steps with your hands resting in your lap.

UJJAYI BREATHING

Ujjayi breathing makes a distinctive "haa" sound and helps you concentrate while practicing standing poses (see pp64–91), as the mind becomes absorbed with the sound of breathing. I find it invaluable in poses such as Tree (see pp76–77) and Half Moon (pp82–83).

This breath is called the Ocean Sounding Breath because the slight constriction in the back of the throat sounds like the hiss of waves in the ocean.

To begin Ujjayi breathing, bring a hand up to your face, the palm open. Imagine that you are holding a pair of glasses and you need to clean them. Fog up the imaginary glasses by exhaling through your mouth onto your hand. Can you feel the warmth and wetness? Can you hear the "haa" sound you make to fog your glasses? Practice this a few times until you feel comfortable with the sound and sensation. Now close your lips and fog the glasses by exhaling through your nostrils. Bring your hand closer to your face to feel the breath from your nostrils. Practice this a few more times. Now imagine that the glasses are located at the back of your skull. Inhale through your nose making the "haa" sound as you fog the glasses. Practice making the "haa" sound a few times, both on the inhale and exhale.

Be mindful to stop if this powerful deep-breathing technique makes you dizzy. After a rest, try again, staying as relaxed and focused as possible.

ALTERNATE NOSTRIL BREATHING

Alternate Nostril breathing sweeps the cobwebs out of your mind. The gentle rhythm of alternating breaths through the left and right nostrils is cleansing and soothing. This technique is the perfect vehicle to take you into Meditation (see pp136–137). Alternate Nostril breathing regulates the right and left hemispheres of the brain and helps to relieve tension headaches and feelings of anxiety. It relaxes the whole body and mind. Use Alternate Nostril breathing at the end of your practice, during meditation.

Note that you will use only the right hand in Alternate Nostril breathing (See Step 1—Step 3, right), even if you are left handed. This technique began in India, where yogis use their left hand for personal hygiene, hence the preference for using the right hand.

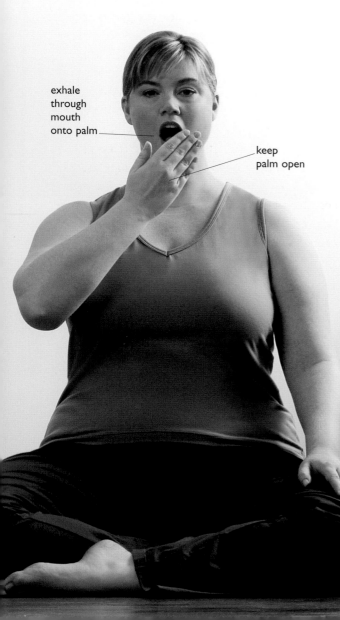

exhale through mouth onto palm

keep palm open

You can feel the deep strength of Ujjayi breathing when you exhale into the palm of your hand. It is the breath of choice for all Standing Poses (see pp64–91).

To begin Alternatate Nostril breathing, follow Steps 1–3, below. As you work, try to keep your fingers as relaxed as possible.

You will find that your breathing is uneven at first, but after a minute or two you will fall into a slow rhythm. I find that, as I practice, my eyes naturally close and I enjoy the sensations of my breathing as it slows down.

Don't try to hold your breath or force it to be slow at first. The breath can be like a tight muscle that relaxes at its own speed in its own time. Get to know your breath and it will become easier for you to observe when you are tensing, holding, or otherwise manipulating it. If you are tense, take some breaths through your mouth. I find this technique particularly helpful whenever I am rapidly becoming fatigued in standing poses (see pp64–91) and want to continue without any muscular tension.

OUR CONSTANT COMPANION

The breath measures out our time on earth. We can live for days without food or water, but we cannot survive for five minutes without breath. We are breathing even when we are not aware of it—while we are sleeping, while we are in the womb. If you are a pregnant woman, you are breathing for your baby. In the West, we measure our life in years. Yogis measure their lives in breaths. To add length to their life, they add length to their breath. Breath is our constant companion. We take it for granted until it is impaired.

Colds, hay fever and other allergies, or sinus troubles can make breathing difficult. When my nose feels stuffy, I practice only Dirgha breathing (see pp26–27). If you're feeling stuffed up try practicing Dirgha in a steamy shower—it feels great. Some plus-size practitioners have sleep apnea, a condition where sleep is interrupted by repeated pauses in breathing. Lack of sleep leaves them feeling chronically exhausted and irritable. If you have this condition, work diligently with Dirgha breathing (see pp26–27) and Alternate Nostril breathing. At the end of your practice, in deep relaxation (see Corpse, pp134–135), use a cushion to keep your torso and head upright, in an elevated position. This will assist your breathing as the elevation helps open your upper air passages.

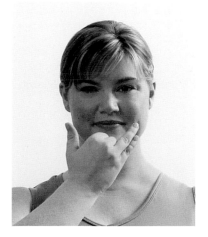

1 Turn your right hand so that your palm is facing you. Fold your index and middle finger into your palm. Take a breath.

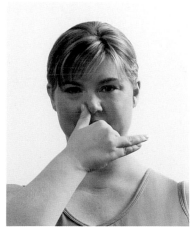

2 Close the side of your right nostril gently with your thumb and exhale through your left nostril. Then inhale.

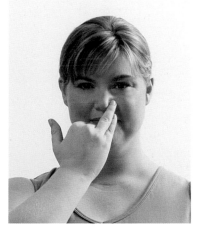

3 Close the side of your left nostril with your ring finger. Exhale and then inhale through your right nostril. Repeat, alternating nostrils.

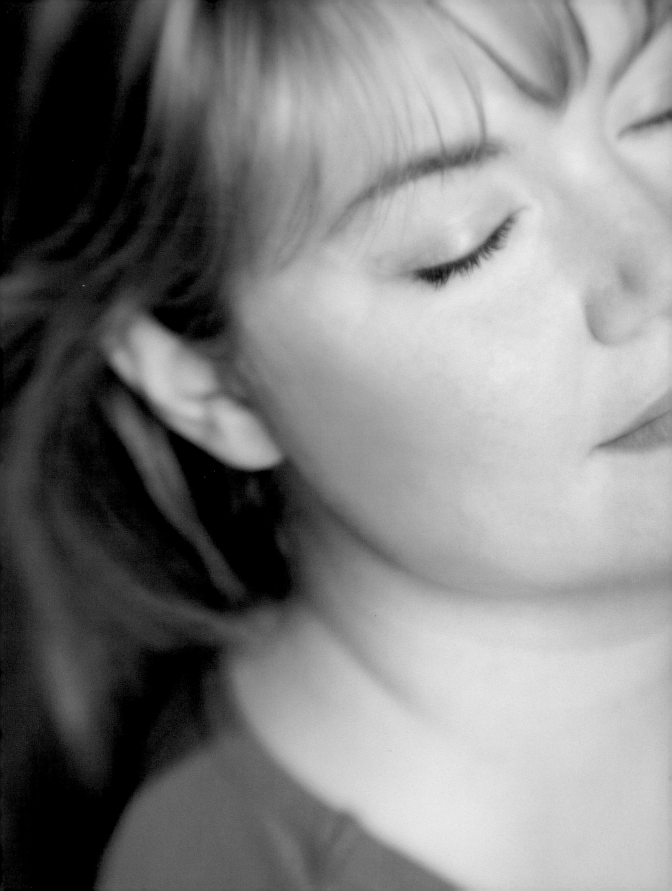

WARM-UPS

Warm-Ups teach us how to coordinate breath with movement, one of the most important skills in yoga. As your body temperature rises with Warm-ups such as Yoga Push-ups and Fire Hydrants, your circulatory system pumps blood to your extremities. Warm-Ups deepen your breath and enliven your muscles with an increase in oxygen—all of which prepares you for the active postures that follow in Standing Poses, Wall Poses and Inversions, Cleansing Poses, and Quiet Poses. Always start your yoga practice with Warm-Ups. I like to warm up beginning with my head and then work down to my legs and feet. Be sure to pay extra attention to any part of your body that feels stiff or achy.

NECK STRETCHES

Warm-ups begin with a series of gentle neck stretches. These stretches activate the entire length of the neck muscles through gentle twisting and releasing. If you choose to try the counter arm stretch on page 33 (please see the Intensifying the Pose box) you will add weight to the neck stretches and increase the pleasurable sensation of these moves.

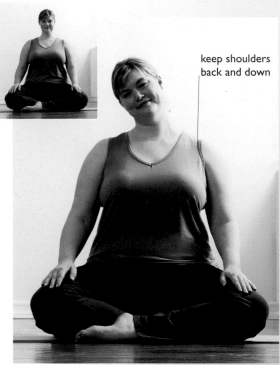

keep shoulders back and down

2 After 5 breaths, on your next exhale, turn your face down and gaze back at the floor behind you. Breathe here for 5 deep breaths. Feel a gentle twist radiate from the base of your neck all the way up into your skull.

1 Sit comfortably with your spine long (inset). Exhaling, drop your right ear over to your right shoulder. Take 5 deep breaths, relaxing your left shoulder back and down. Feel a long line of energy running up and down the left side of your neck.

drop your
jaw, open
your mouth

3 After 5 breaths, on your next inhale, turn your face up to the ceiling. On the exhale open your mouth and let out a big "ahhhhh," sighing out any tension.

4 Breathing easily, roll your head around in a circle. If you notice any discomfort, back off and make the circle smaller. Circle in both directions. When you feel complete, repeat the series on the other side.

INTENSIFYING THE POSE

To generate more sensation in Neck Stretches reach your arm away from your head. Feel the stretch from your fingertips all the way up your arm into the base of your skull. Perform all the steps with your arm outstretched. Then repeat on the other side.

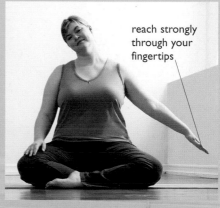

reach strongly through your fingertips

SUN BREATHS

As your arms mimic the rising and setting of the sun's rays, you will coordinate breath and movement in Sun Breaths. The intercostal muscles between your ribs stretch, your lungs expand, and all the components of deep breathing are awakened. As you lift and lower your arms, imagine that you are moving them through mud, feeling the resistance as you go. Let your inhaled and exhaled breaths dictate the speed of your arms, matching your movement and breath as best as you can. After several repetitions this will get easier to coordinate as your breath slows down naturally.

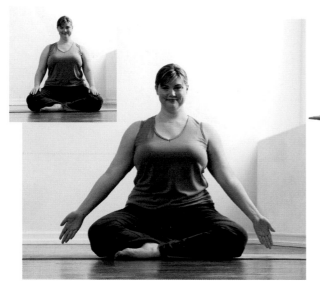

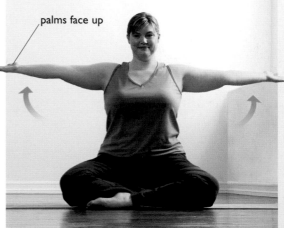

palms face up

1 Begin in a simple seated posture (inset), then lower your arms to the floor, palms out. Roll your thumbs back and down to really stretch the insides of your arms.

Awaken the body as you awaken the breath.

2 Inhale as you sweep your arms up overhead. Move slowly, inhale slowly. Keep reaching out through your fingertips.

3 Continue inhaling, sweeping your arms up to the sky. As you reach up, feel the connection of your buttocks to the floor.

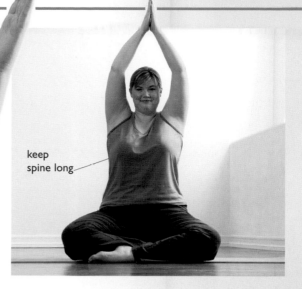

keep
spine long

4 At the top of your inhale, let your palms touch. Then begin your exhale as you sweep your arms slowly out and down.

palms
face down

5 At shoulder level turn your palms down. Pause at the bottom of the exhale when your fingertips touch the floor and then inhale again as your arms sweep up for another round. Practice 5 rounds of Sun Breaths.

SEATED TWIST

Yoga twists are powerful internal cleansers. When you twist, your movement squeezes the muscles and internal organs on the side into which you are twisting. As you hold and breathe, the blood supply to that area is slowed down. When you release, freshly oxygenated blood shoots into the muscles, bathing the organs on that side.

MODIFYING THE POSE

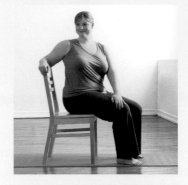

You can use the back of a chair to help you in the twist. Sit forward, keeping your back straight. Be careful not to over-twist by gripping and pulling on the chair.

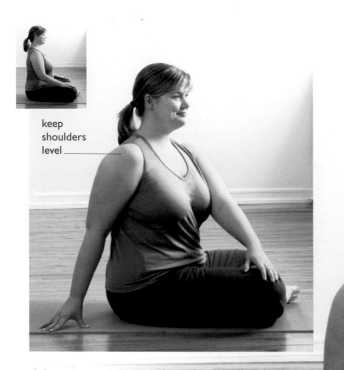

keep shoulders level

press up

1 Start in a simple seated posture (inset). Exhale as you place your left hand on your right knee and your right hand behind you on the floor.

2 Inhale, pressing up through the crown of your head. Exhale and twist, starting the movement at the base of your spine. Continue for 5 breaths, each breath taking you deeper into the twist. Then untwist, rest, and repeat on the other side.

ROCKING LEGS

Rocking provides a gradual warm-up for the hips and buttocks. Choose a hand position that feels comfortable for you—pointing your hands either in toward your body or away. Keep your back long and your chest lifted as you rock. Let the speed of your breath match the speed of your movements side to side.

INTENSIFYING THE POSE

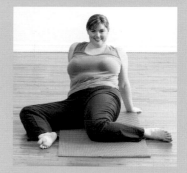

Begin to move your feet further apart to intensify the stretch in your hips. As you warm up you can separate them even further.

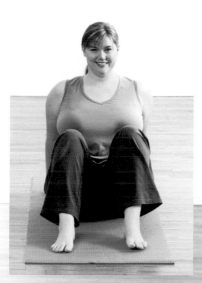

1 Sit with your feet flat on the floor in front of you, knees bent. Place your hands behind you for support.

2 Exhale and drop your knees down to the right. Inhale as you come back up to the center and exhale as you drop your legs down to the left. Repeat five times on each side.

roll hip up and over

drop knee to floor

ANKLE ROLLS AND MASSAGE

This warm-up bathes the ankle in synovial fluid—a substance that lubricates all the movable joints in the body, much the way engine oil bathes all the the movable parts in a car. Unlike the heart, which pumps blood through our bodies, the movement of synovial fluid is stimulated only by actual physical movement. This is why your feet may feel stiff and inflexible when you first wake up, or after prolonged sitting in a car or airplane.

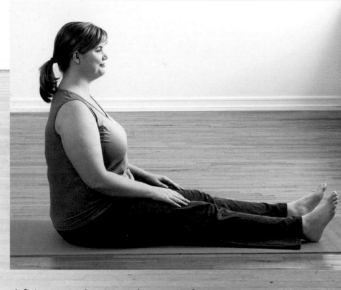

1 Bring your legs straight out in front of you. Sit up tall, with the sitz bones of your pelvis anchored to the floor.

2 Draw your left foot up, resting it on your right thigh.

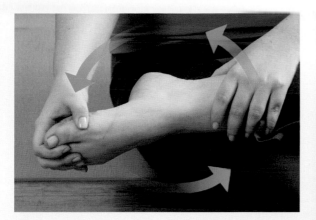

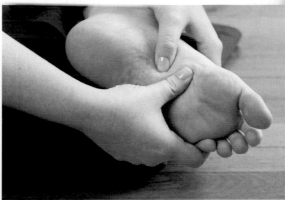

3 Taking hold of your toes, slowly circle your foot as you breathe in and out. Be sure to go counterclockwise, too, when you are ready.

4 Walk your thumbs up and down the arch of your foot. Feel free to use any other massage technique that feels delicious. Enjoy!

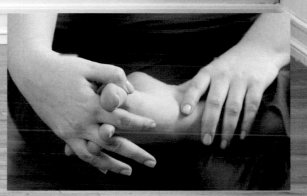

5 Place your fingers between your toes to spread them wide. Bend your toes back and forth several times. Now switch legs and repeat.

foot should be above or below kneecap, not on it

ROCK THE BABY

Rocking your legs warms up the the hips and glutes (the large muscles of the buttocks). Remember to keep your back long and your heart lifted as you rock. Focus on bringing each leg up to you, rather than bending down to meet it. I'm lucky enough to have very open hips so sometimes I even kiss my toes! This cracks up my students every time. A wise yogi once said, "Yoga is too important to take seriously." Great advice for yoga and for life, don't you agree?

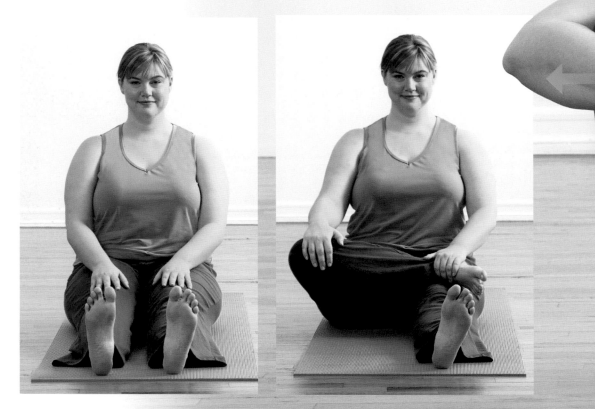

1 In a seated position, bring your legs straight out in front of you. Flex your feet and enjoy the hamstring stretch.

2 Draw your right foot up, resting it on your left thigh. Your foot should be positioned either above or below the knee.

keep spine long

3 Pick up your bent right leg and cradle it with both arms, drawing it in toward your chest. As you breathe, gently rock your leg from side to side, making the movement larger as you go. After several rounds, repeat on the other side.

hug leg into body

INTENSIFYING THE POSE

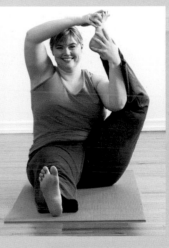

If you have very open hips, you can try lifting your foot higher to intensify the stretch. Remember to keep your pelvis anchored and your chest lifted so that you don't hunch forward in an attempt to lift the foot too high.

GENTLE STARFISH

A strong set of abdominals is vital for lower back health. Concentrate on initiating movement on the exhale so that your abdominals contract with the effort. As always, listen to your internal cues. If you feel any discomfort, back off and take a brief rest. You will get stronger steadily. When I practice the pose correctly my belly shakes like crazy. If this happens to you, don't worry—it's a signal that your abdominals are strengthening. Don't try to squelch this natural release of energy. Let your belly shake!

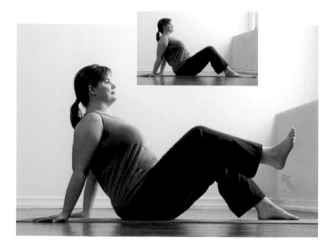

1 Sit with your hands behind you, palms down, fingertips pointing away from you. Your feet are flat on the floor, knees bent (inset). Exhaling, draw your right leg into your body. Inhale. Then, exhaling, press your foot away. Repeat 5 times.

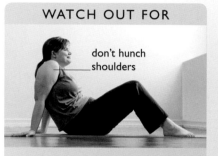

WATCH OUT FOR

don't hunch shoulders

Keep your chest lifted, your head high, and your neck long. Be mindful not to hunch. Slouching deactives the abdominals and puts too much strain on the lower back.

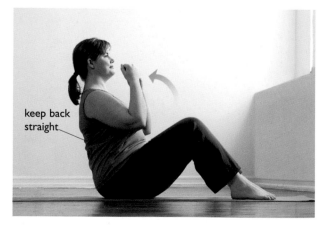

keep back straight

2 Put your feet back down on the floor and inhale. Exhale and draw your arms into your body. Inhale. Exhale and rock back a few inches. Repeat 5 times.

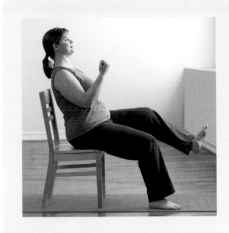

MODIFYING THE POSE

Like all seated Warm-ups, Gentle Starfish can be done in a chair. This is the best version for beginners or for anyone who has lower back sensitivity. In Step 2 be sure to always leave one foot on the floor. Sit tall and don't slouch into the back of the chair.

keep foot flexed

lift chest

3 Exhaling, draw in your right leg and left arm. Inhale. Exhale and press your right foot away as you rock back just an inch or two. Repeat 5 times. Be sure to alternate and repeat on the other side for 5 repetitions.

VIGOROUS STARFISH

After you have mastered Gentle Starfish (see pp42–43) you will be ready for a bigger abdominal challenge. Vigorous Starfish coordinates the movement of both arms and legs simultaneously, and is therefore more challenging. The movement starts from your core, so concentrate on initiating from your belly. Keep your back long and chest lifted as you work. Most importantly, breathe, using strong exhales on each movement for maximum support.

CAUTION
Avoid both Gentle Starfish (pp42–43) and Vigorous Starfish if you have:
• back pain
• disk or neck injury
• osteoporosis
• hernia or recent abdominal injury

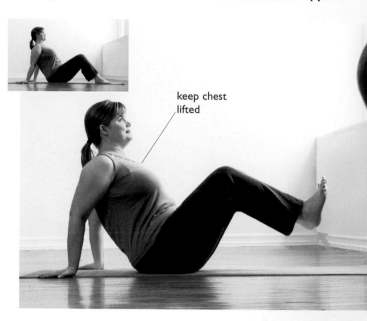

keep chest lifted

keep back flat

1 Sit with your hands behind you, palms down, fingertips pointing away from you. Your feet should be flat on the floor, knees bent (inset). Exhaling, bring both feet in toward your chest. Inhale. Then, exhaling, press them away from you. Repeat 5 times.

Notice how your mind starts to chatter during vigorous moves. This is a good sign that you are becoming more involved in your practice.

2 Exhaling, bring your arms into your body. Your feet should be flat on the floor. Inhale. Exhaling, rock back a few inches. Repeat 5 times, keeping your back long.

INTENSIFYING THE POSE

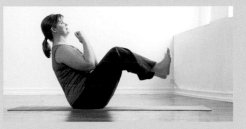

1. To intensify the pose, move all your limbs simultaneously. Inhale. Exhaling, bring your arms and legs into your body, curling up into a ball. See the second part of the intensifier, below.

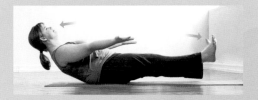

2. Inhale, then exhale, as you reach outward with your arms and legs floating a few inches above the floor. Inhale. Exhaling, curl back up, squeezing your navel into your spine. Repeat 5 times.

TABLE TOP

Table Top is the first held balancing move in Warm-Ups. It strengthens the back, torso, and buttocks as it stretches the front of the body. Notice that as soon as you start to concentrate you immediately hold your breath. It's funny how we think this will help keep us balanced and aloft in Table Top, when the opposite is true. Deep Dirgha breathing (see pp26–27) will power you through this warm-up and prevent your arms and legs from cramping.

> **MEGA TIP**
>
> This is a great pose for strengthening your glutes. In Step 2 squeeze your buttocks as you focus on stretching the surface of your body into a level table top.

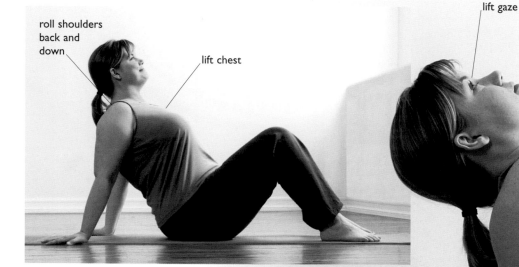

roll shoulders back and down

lift chest

lift gaze

don't clench jaw

keep elbows soft, don't lock them

1 Sit with your feet flat on the floor, hands behind you, fingers facing away from you. Keep your heart lifted and inhale.

2 Exhale and squeeze your buttocks, lifting your torso and forming a table top with the front of your body. Breathe here for 5 deep Dirgha breaths.

MODIFYING THE POSE

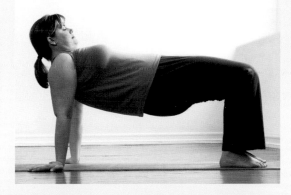 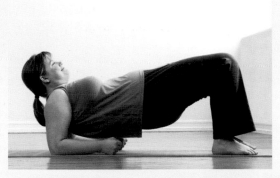

The head is heavy, and it takes neck strength to dip it back in the full pose. If you feel discomfort, alternate looking up and down to build neck strength. Be mindful not to hunch your shoulders.

If you have carpal tunnel syndrome in the wrists or any other wrist injury or sensitivity, practice Table Top with your forearms on the floor. Keep squeezing your buttocks to help lift your torso.

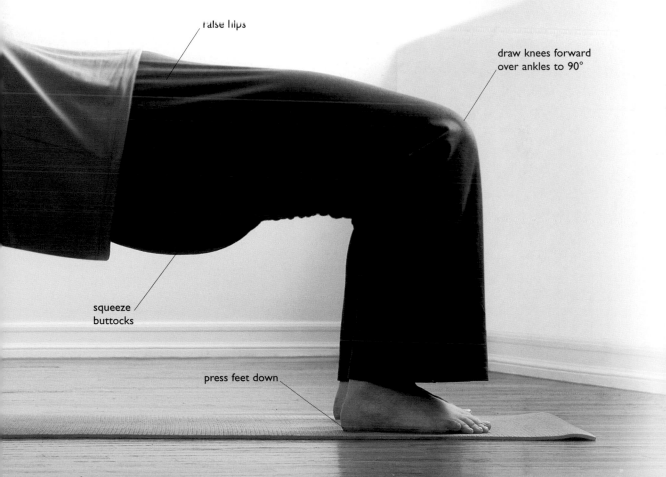

raise hips

draw knees forward over ankles to 90°

squeeze buttocks

press feet down

BODY ARCH

This graceful moving arch synchronizes breath with movement and stretches the entire length of the torso. If you feel knee discomfort when you arch up, place a folded blanket beneath your knee. The shoulder circles at the top of the arch in Step 4 use gravity to warm up the shoulder joint.

> **MEGA TIP**
> If your hips are really lifted in Step 4, you should be able to come up onto your fingertips. Squeeze your buttocks to fly up.

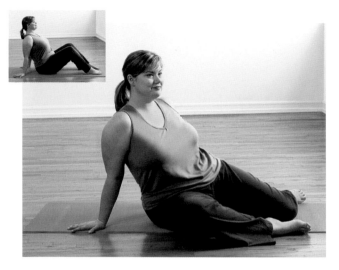

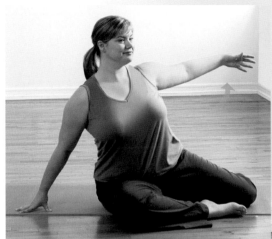

1 Begin in a seated position, knees bent, hands behind your back, fingers pointing away from you (inset). Flop your legs over to the right side.

2 Inhale your left arm up to shoulder height. Let the inhale help you come up onto the fingertips of your right hand.

3 Exhaling, swing your arm across your body, twisting as you go. Tap you back shoulder with your fingertips and then swing back to Step 2 as you inhale. Repeat 5 times.

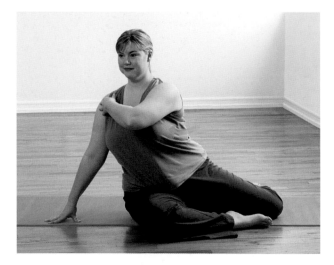

4 Now exhale and swing your arm
up overhead as you squeeze your
buttocks and lift your hips up off the
floor. Maintain the squeeze as you circle
the lifted arm for 5 deep breaths. Lower
and repeat on the other side.

squeeze
buttocks

keep weight off
supporting hand
by squeezing
buttocks

CAT AND DOG TILTS

Gentle forward and back bends awaken the spine and promote disk health. The tilts in Cat and Dog extend all the way from the tip of your skull to the bottom of your tailbone, so be mindful to tilt your pelvis, too. Be careful not to overarch your neck and compress the cervical spine. Let the movement start from the center of your belly and then ripple through the length of your spine. This is similar to the movement principle in Gentle Starfish (see pp42–43).

see pp42–43

> **MEGA TIP**
>
> Start with small movements and then let your tilts get larger as you deepen your breath. Start at 20 percent and then gradually go to 100 percent.

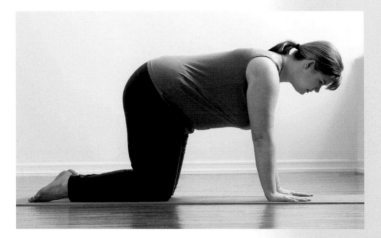

1 Begin on your hands and knees. If you feel any discomfort, place a folded yoga mat or blanket under your knees for cushioning. Take 5 breaths here and feel the movement of your belly rising as you inhale. As you exhale, your navel moves in toward your spine.

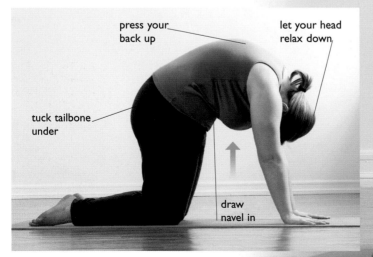

press your back up

let your head relax down

tuck tailbone under

draw navel in

2 Exhale, drawing your navel in as you press up strongly through your upper back. Your forehead and pubic bone should draw together so that your entire back forms a beautiful C curve. At the end of the exhale immediately move into step 3.

Little kids can't resist this playful move.
I love to teach it to them, complete with
meows in "Cat" and woofs in "Dog."

3 Inhale as you reverse the movements.
Press your chest forward and up while
your sacrum tilts up to the ceiling. Enjoy the
stretch in your belly. Repeat these movements
10 times without stopping. Match the speed
of your tilting to your breath.

gaze up

tailbone
lifts up

keep shoulders
back and down

MODIFYING THE POSE

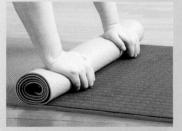

If your wrists hurt, roll up the
edge of a yoga mat and grip it for
added cushioning and to reduce
the angle of wrist flexion.

TABLE BALANCE

Table Balance strengthens your buttocks, stomach, and legs as well as improving your balance. Regular practice with deep Dirgha breathing (see pp26–27) will keep your lower back happy. If your knees do not tolerate kneeling in this warm-up, use a folded blanket or a small pillow for padding. Knees don't get "tougher" or more muscular with use. Pamper them!

MODIFYING THE POSE

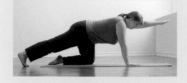

If balancing on fewer than three points is a challenge for you in this pose, keep both feet on the floor. Don't worry about achieving balance the "hard" way.

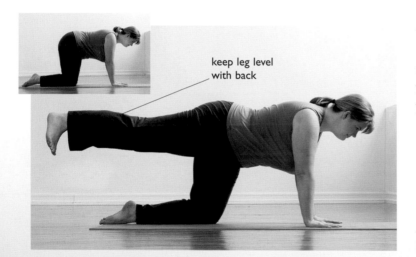

keep leg level with back

1 Begin on your hands and knees (inset). Exhaling, lift your right leg up to hip height, flexing your foot. Breathe as you keep your hips level for two breaths.

2 Inhale and exhale, lifting your left arm to hip height. Hold for 5 breaths as your extended arm and leg reach in opposite directions. Now switch and repeat on the other side.

keep hips rolled down and level

keep back flat

KIDNEY SQUEEZE

This spinal warm-up with side-to-side movement is the natural complement to Cat and Dog Tilts (see pp50–51). Be mindful to keep your gaze directed at the floor at all times so that you squeeze side to side without overtwisting your neck. Study the photo in Step 2 and you will see that both your hips and shoulders move together. As you practice, try to feel them squeezing together to make the C curve.

> **MEGA TIP**
>
> For a good illustration of exactly how Kidney Squeeze works, take a look at the overhead photograph in Step 2 to see the C curve in action.

1 Begin on your hands and knees. If you feel any discomfort in your knees, cushion them with a folded yoga mat or a blanket.

2 Exhale and shift your hips and shoulders to the right in a C curve, squeezing out all the air. Without stopping, inhale, then move back to the center and exhale to the left side. Repeat the move, going side to side, 10 times.

see the
C curve

keep gaze
down

feel a gentle
stretch in the
nonsqueezing side

FIRE HYDRANTS

Fire Hydrants build lots of heat in the muscles of the legs and buttocks. You'll understand why we call them *warm*-ups! Have you heard the saying that women generally have stronger lower bodies than upper bodies? I coasted along on that bit of information for quite a while and didn't really challenge my lower body until I began practicing Fire Hydrants regularly.

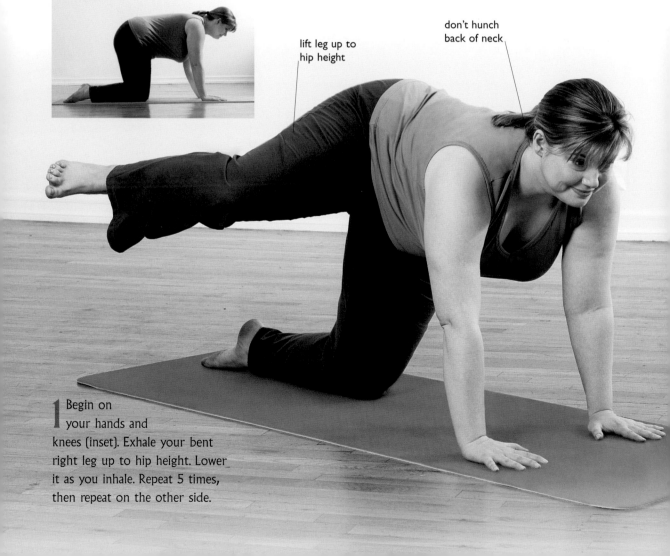

lift leg up to hip height

don't hunch back of neck

1 Begin on your hands and knees (inset). Exhale your bent right leg up to hip height. Lower it as you inhale. Repeat 5 times, then repeat on the other side.

HIP CIRCLES

Hip Circles move the spine in a fluid circle after the up/down flexion of Cat and Dog Tilts (see pp50–51) and the side-to-side C curve of Kidney Squeeze (see p53). As I warm up in Hip Circles, I move faster and faster, finally letting go with an audible, exhaled "haaa"—a great way to release bottled up tension.

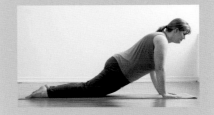
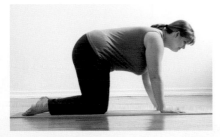

keep shoulders relaxed

1 Begin on your hands and knees (inset). Breathe slowly and circle your hips around and around. After several cycles, circle your hips in the other direction.

YOGA PUSH-UPS

These gentle push-ups strengthen the triceps and pectoral muscles. For many of us with heavy chests, strong pecs and backs enable us to carry our weight and stand tall. Start with small push-ups, then gradually make the movement larger as you go. If your knees are uncomfortable, place a folded blanket or pillow under them for cushioning.

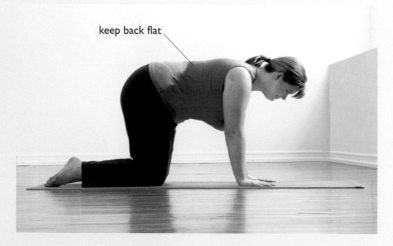

keep back flat

1 Begin on your hands and knees. Deepen your breath slowly. The push-up is less intense if you keep your weight back over your heels and more intense if you bring your weight forward over your hands.

INTENSIFYING THE POSE

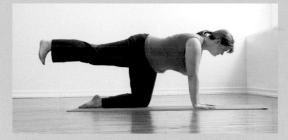

Begin on your hands and knees. Reach one leg back behind you, keeping your foot in line with your torso. Notice that the hip of the active leg wants to roll up to the ceiling. Resist this as you level off your hips.

Now do the push-up while raising the extended leg. Keep your hips level. You can use my personal mantra for inspiration here: "Way to go rock star!" This fires up my spirit while the pose heats up the rest of me.

keep
back flat

2 Inhale and then exhale, drawing in your abdominals and lowering your chest toward the floor, elbows dropping straight back behind you. Inhale and press back up. Repeat for 5 to 10 breaths.

drop elbows straight back, in line with the sides of your body

put a cushion under your knees if you are uncomfortable kneeling

CHILD'S POSE

Child's Pose is a touchstone to come back to whenever you feel overwhelmed or fatigued during your practice. Curling your body into a fetal position, your head below your heart, is deeply soothing for the nervous system. For the animal self, when the front of the body is covered, the internal organs are protected. For the thinking self, the increased blood flow to the head is beneficial for brain function. For the secret self, the head below the heart symbolizes the submission of the intellect to the emotions. In many cultures a deep bow is a posture for prayer and reverence.

breathe into
your back

spread knees

reach fingers
toward end of mat

MODIFYING THE POSE

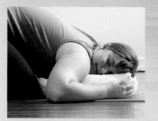

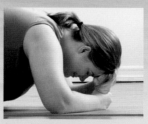

For extra support and comfort in this pose, hug a big pillow or a cushion. If it hurts to kneel, place a folded blanket or a small pillow under your knees.

If your forehead does not reach the floor you can make little fists, one on top of the other and rest your forehead on them.

1 Drop your hips back toward your heels, spreading your knees wide enough to accommodate your chest and belly. Reach your fingers toward the top of your mat. Rest your forehead on the mat and close your eyes. Hold the pose for 10 deep breaths, breathing into your back.

UNDERARM STRETCH

Underarm Stretch may look like a static pose—but in reality your hips and hands never stop moving. The stretch provides a delightful opening for the backs of the arms and the armpits. Try it before any activity that involves arm strength such as carrying a toddler or heavy shopping bags. Don't forget to keep crawling your fingers forward on the mat as you sit back on your buttocks.

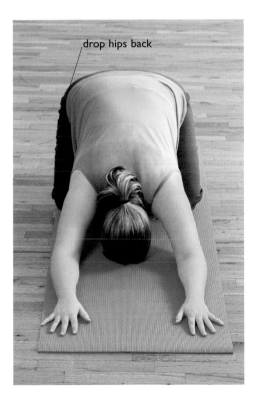

drop hips back

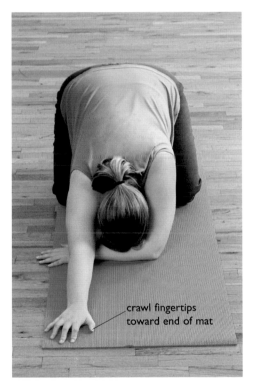

crawl fingertips toward end of mat

1 Start in Child's pose (see opposite), dropping your hips back toward your heels, your belly and chest comfortably positioned between your legs. Your forehead should rest comfortably on the mat, your arms extended forward.

2 Exhaling, draw your left arm back behind your right elbow. Crawl your right fingertips away from you toward the end of the mat. Keep the back of your right arm in front of your left hand. After five breaths, change sides. Repeat with the other arm.

MINDFUL STANDING

I injured my lower back a while ago picking up a heavy load of laundry incorrectly, and the warm-ups you've learned played a big part in my recovery. As I was healing, resting on the floor in Legs up the Wall (see pp104–105) with an ice pack, I realized that sooner or later I would have to get up. The thought of standing was intimidating—one forward bend and I'd be in pain. Mindful Standing is not a pose, it's a transitional move that was created out of necessity. I needed a way to use the power of my legs to propel me upright without bending my spine. Mindful Standing will show you how to get off the floor without straining your back. All the steps flow together and are meant to be practiced in a fluid manner. If you need to rest in any step, do so.

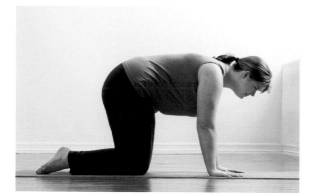

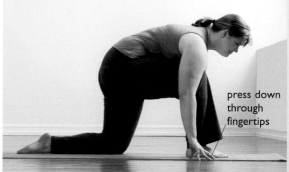

press down
through
fingertips

1 Begin on your hands and knees, your back flat, palms down. Give your buttocks a strong squeeze. Breathe here, feeling the movement in your belly.

2 Inhale and then exhale, bringing your right leg forward between your hands. Your knee should be under your armpit to keep your breasts and belly free. Come up onto your fingertips and exhale.

3 Walk one hand and then the other up onto the bent leg. Make sure your back is flat.

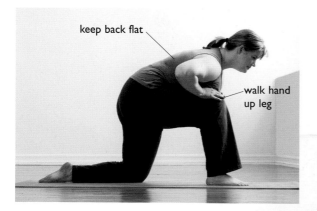

keep back flat

walk hand up leg

curl toes under

Mindfulness means paying attention to what you feel, where you are, and how you move. Bring this mindful quality to every move in your practice.

4 Keep walking your hands up your bent leg until your torso is upright and you are looking straight ahead. Curl the toes of your left foot under, to prepare for standing.

keep back straight

press hands into top of thigh for support

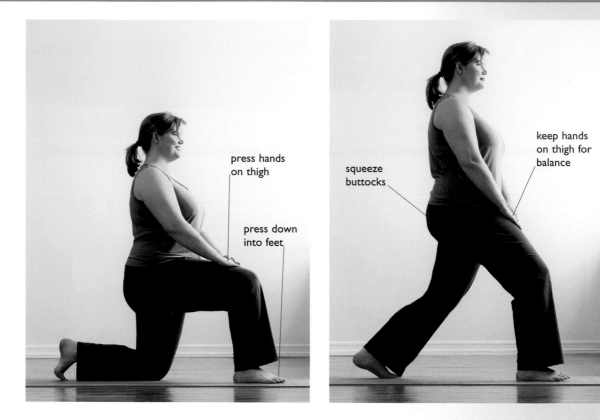

press hands on thigh

press down into feet

squeeze buttocks

keep hands on thigh for balance

5 Shift your weight slightly forward to the foot in front of you. Get ready to come up by pressing down into your feet. Take a breath.

6 Exhale as you squeeze your buttocks vigorously and come up. You can keep your hands on your leg or out to the side for more balance.

Mindful Standing also works in reverse whenever you need to go down to the floor from standing.

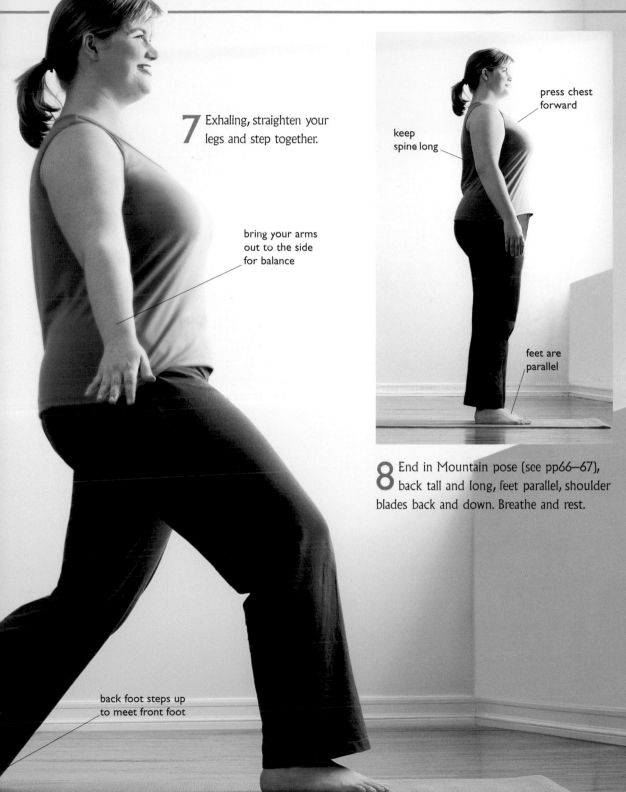

7 Exhaling, straighten your legs and step together.

bring your arms out to the side for balance

press chest forward

keep spine long

feet are parallel

8 End in Mountain pose (see pp66–67), back tall and long, feet parallel, shoulder blades back and down. Breathe and rest.

back foot steps up to meet front foot

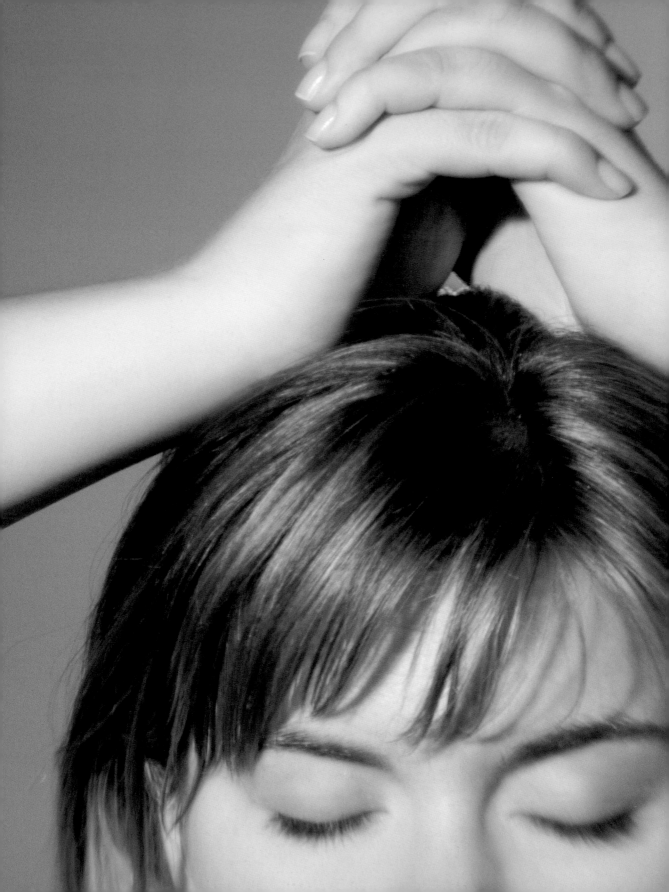

STANDING POSES

Standing poses build strength and flexibility in the
lower body. We begin in Mountain pose, learning
how to stand tall with grace. Warrior, Goddess,
Eagle, and Awkward pose all involve squatting or
lunging to strengthen our legs and hips. Tree and
Half Moon heighten our sense of balance. All of
the poses develop symmetry on both sides of the
body. Practice all Standing poses utilizing Ujjayi
breathing (see p28). If you find that Ujjayi is a
strain, try breathing in through your nostrils and
then opening your mouth to exhale. I find this
trick helpful when I am in a pose that is difficult
for me and I begin to hold my breath.
Remember to practice strong, not strained.

MOUNTAIN

I didn't slouch as a little ballerina in grade school. I wanted all eyes to be on me as I danced. However, when I developed breasts I felt that the eyes looking at me were coming from a different place. I started slouching then and kept slouching until I walked into a yoga class in college. The teacher created a safe space where I could stand tall without comment, without sexual energy, without judgment. It freed me from the slouch.

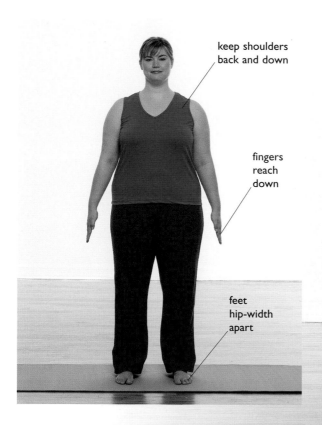

palms face each other

keep shoulders back and down

fingers reach down

feet hip-width apart

1 After finding your perfect hip-width by hopping in place (see General Alignment, pp16–17), align your feet parallel. Reach down through your fingertips.

MEGA TIP

Try Mountain pose with your eyes closed. Let yourself make micro-movements to stay balanced. Use your inner awareness to sense where you are.

Mountains are majestic, beautiful, and awe-inspiring. When you enter this pose, imagine that you are a mighty mountain, whose peaks reach up into the clouds.

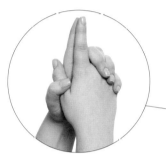

Temple position

2 Inhaling, sweep your arms overhead, fingers reaching up to the sky. Hold for 5 deep Ujjayi breaths. Then lower and relax your arms.

press down into soles of feet

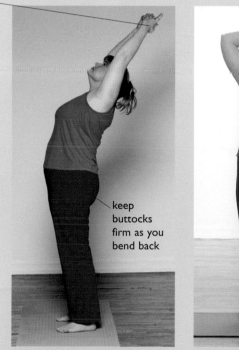

MODIFYING THE POSE

keep buttocks firm as you bend back

To Intensify the pose: After Step 2 bring your hands into Temple position (see inset). Inhaling, reach up, and, exhaling, slowly arch backward as if you were drawing a line straight back behind you on the ceiling with your fingertips.

As an alternative intensification of the pose: If you cannot bring your arms straight overhead with your hands in Temple without hunching your shoulders, you can bend your elbows and simply rest your hands on the crown of your head.

WARRIOR 1

Across cultures, victorious athletes and weekend warriors throw their arms up and jump for joy upon victory. This feeling of ecstasy is distilled into Warrior 1. The dynamic lunge strengthens the feet, legs, and hips while improving balance. If you are able to lift your arms into a big V you will also work your back and shoulders. Try the modification with two chairs for support on shaky days or if balancing is a challenge.

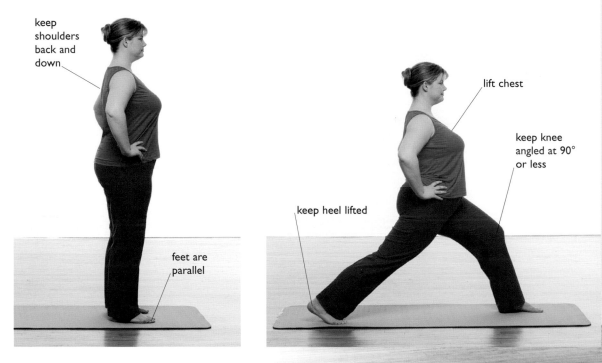

keep shoulders back and down

feet are parallel

lift chest

keep knee angled at 90° or less

keep heel lifted

1 Stand at the front of your mat with feet hip-width apart. Inhale deeply and place your hands on your hips.

2 Exhale as you lunge back with your right leg, heel lifted. Keep your feet and hips forward. Don't let your right hip roll out to the side.

arms make
V shape

MODIFYING THE POSE

Using two chairs for support is a good way to feel confident in the lunge. Make sure the chairs are sturdy and of equal height. When you step together to exit the pose, try not to lean heavily on the chairs.

hips face
forward

3 Inhale your arms up into a big V, fingers reaching to the sky. Gaze straight ahead and take 5 deep Ujjayi breaths. Reverse the steps to exit the pose, and repeat on the other side.

WARRIOR 2

The warrior in this second variation is poised in the midst of battle. She stands balanced directly over her center of gravity, looking out towards the horizon like an archer drawing a bow taut (see Step 3). The key to the pose lies in keeping your torso over your hips at all times. Don't be too eager to reach forward or lunge deeper. As you gain strength in your practice you will simply take a wider stance for a deeper lunge. The spirit of the poised warrior is expressed in the balanced relationship of torso over hips.

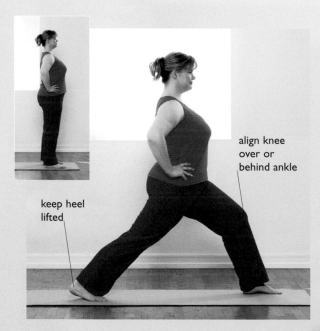

keep heel lifted

align knee over or behind ankle

pelvis faces forward

1 Stand at the front of your mat with feet hip-width apart, hands on your hips (inset). Exhaling, lunge your right leg back to a comfortable distance.

2 Inhale. Exhale and turn your right foot out 45°. Allow your pelvis to follow the turn of the back foot and face out as shown.

back foot turned out 45°

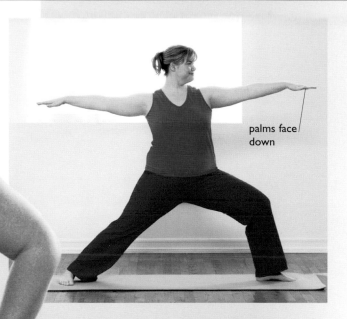

palms face down

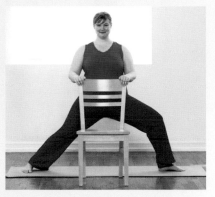

MODIFYING THE POSE

If balancing is difficult for you, practice with a chair for support. Anyone with sensitive knees will enjoy this modification. When you enter and exit the pose try not to lean heavily on the chair.

3 Keeping your lower body still, inhale and raise your arms up to shoulder height. Gaze straight ahead at the hand in front of you and begin deep Ujjayi breathing. Hold the pose for 5 breaths, then reverse the steps and repeat on the other side.

INTENSIFYING THE POSE

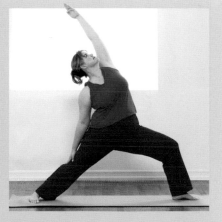

align knee over or behind ankle

Add a gentle back bend after Step 3 for a deep stretch up your torso. Inhale your forward arm up to the sky as your back hand floats down your extended leg. Gaze at your raised hand and breathe in the stretch.

5-POINTED STAR

5-Pointed Star looks like Leonardo Da Vinci's famous study of male anatomy, the sketch of the Vitruvian Man. Enjoy the long lines of your limbs radiating from your center as you press the floor away with your feet and press the walls away with your hands. Press the ceiling away with the crown of your head.

keep arms level with shoulders

hips face forward

1 Begin in Mountain pose, arms at your sides, feet parallel at your body's natural hip width.

2 Inhaling, step out wide as you sweep your arms up to shoulder height, palms parallel to the floor and aligned over your feet. Hold for 5–10 deep Ujjayi breaths. To exit the pose, bring your feet together in a heel-toe motion or flow into Goddess (see opposite page).

GODDESS

If 5-Pointed Star captures the lines of male anatomy, Goddess expresses the curvy angles of a woman in a deep squat. Enjoy surrendering to gravity as you sink down and are drawn toward the earth. Across the world, many women choose to labor while squatting, letting gravity work with them in delivering their babies. Squatting improves blood flow and is a natural treatment for varicose veins and poor circulation in the calves and feet.

> **MEGA TIP**
>
> Be mindful to keep your back vertical at all times to avoid strain in your knees and lower back.

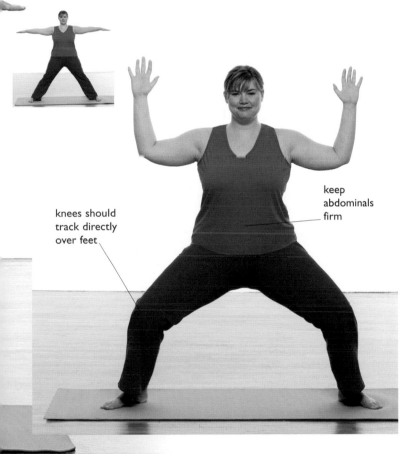

knees should track directly over feet

keep abdominals firm

Toddlers can squat all day long looking for pebbles on the beach. Recapture that freedom when you practice Goddess.

MODIFYING THE POSE

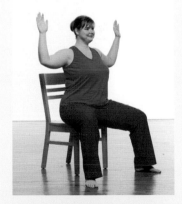

If squatting without support is uncomfortable because of balance or strength issues, remain seated on the edge of a chair and pulse your arms as you breathe.

1 Begin in 5-Pointed Star (inset). Exhaling, squat down as if you had a heavy weight attached to your tailbone. Bend your elbows deeply and spread your fingers wide, palms facing out. Inhale back up into 5-Pointed Star. Repeat 5–10 times, squatting a little deeper each time.

QUARTER MOON

Just like Kidney Squeeze in Warm-ups (see p53), Quarter Moon gently squeezes the sides of the waist, a move that flushes the kidneys with a fresh supply of blood when the squeeze is released. In Quarter Moon, imagine that you are arching over a waist–high fence as you lean up and over into the arch. Let the hip you are arching away from press out to the side. Keep your feet grounded as best as you can. Let your arms frame your face while you maintain a long neck.

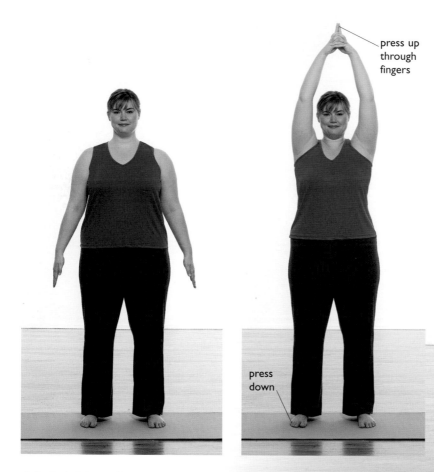

press up through fingers

press hip out to the right

press down

1 Begin in Mountain pose, arms at your sides, feet parallel at your body's natural hip width.

2 Inhaling, bring your arms up overhead, shoulder width apart, hands in Temple position.

3 Exhaling, arch over to your left as you press your right hip strongly away from you to the right. Squeeze your buttocks. Reach through your fingertips. Inhale to come back to center and exhale to arch over to the other side. Repeat 5–10 cycles.

I used to imagine myself arching over a barbed wire fence in this pose because I was raised on a farm. Trust me, you don't want to lean on one!

MODIFYING THE POSE

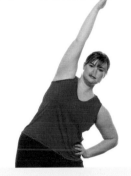

If you have lower back pain or a shoulder injury that prevents you from lifting both arms at once, place your left hand on your left hip and inhale your right arm up as you arch. Repeat 5–10 cycles.

WATCH OUT FOR

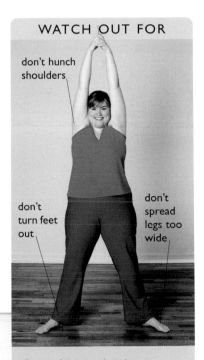

don't hunch shoulders

don't turn feet out

don't spread legs too wide

Be careful not to hunch your shoulders. Your feet should be parallel to each other, not splayed. Don't forget about hopping in place to find your natural hip width.

TREE

Trees appear to be completely still on a calm day, but beneath the earth, their roots grow downward. In this posture, you can embody the dynamic up-and-down motion of a growing tree. Root your standing leg into the ground, reach upward with your fingertips toward the sun, and let your breath move through your body as sap flows through a tree. You can modify the pose by using a wall for support. Many beautiful saplings are trained to grow up a stake until they are strong enough to stay up on their own.

> **MEGA TIP**
>
> In yoga class, focus on a spot on the wall in front of you—not on the back of another yoga student. If she falls over, you will too! Pick a spot that doesn't move.

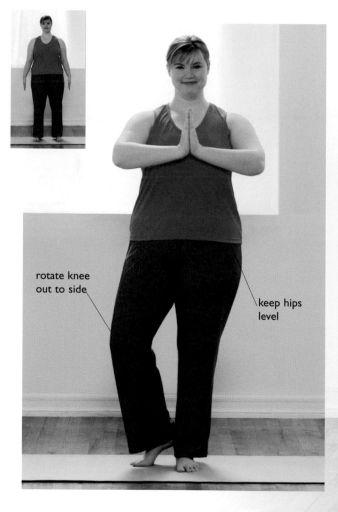

rotate knee out to side

keep hips level

bring back knee

1 Begin in Mountain pose, hands at your sides (inset). Inhaling, bring your hands up to prayer position over your heart and rotate your right leg out to the side, resting your heel on your left ankle. Take five deep breaths as you sway in the posture. Gaze at a point in front of you and breathe to that point.

press up through
crown of head

MODIFYING THE POSE

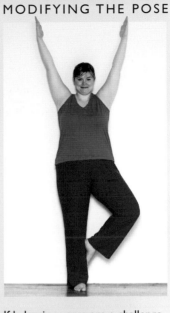

keep chest
lifted

keep hips level
and tailbone
slightly tucked

If balancing poses are a challenge,
you can practice Tree pose against
a wall for support during Step 2.
As you turn out your bent, lifted
leg press it into the wall.

2 Inhaling, draw your right foot
up your left leg, resting it on
the inside of your left calf. Sweep your
arms up to the sky, fingertips stretching
upward like the branches of a tree. Feel
yourself simultaneously reaching down and
up, as you breathe for 5 deep Ujjayi breaths.
Then lower and repeat on the other side.

keep heel on calf,
not on side of knee

TRIANGLE

I discovered the essence of Triangle on a New York City subway. If you have ever caught the commuter rush early in the morning, when every strap or pole is occupied, you may have been left standing with nothing to hold on to. As the train hurtles down the track, the only way you can keep from falling is to take a wide stance and squeeze your inner thighs.

MEGA TIP

If you need to hold on to your shin with your hand in Step 3, you have deactivated your abdominals. When I do the pose, as shown, my stomach shakes like crazy because it is working!

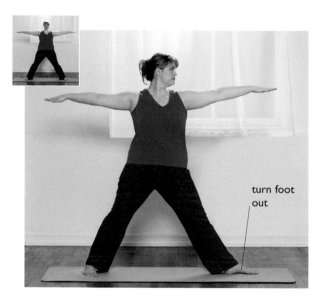

turn foot out

1 Begin in 5-Pointed Star (inset). Inhaling, turn your left foot out 90° as you gaze straight ahead at your outstretched left fingertips.

roll hip up and back

squeeze thigh muscles to bone

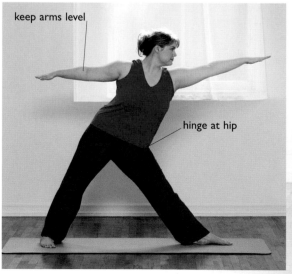

keep arms level

hinge at hip

2 Exhaling, reach toward the front of your mat through your left fingertips and hinge at the hips. Imagine that your arms are resting on a table. Don't let them drop to the floor. If they drop, you have worked beyond the strength of your abdominals.

gaze at fingertips or down at the floor

roll armpit up and back

I used to get frustrated that I'd never get this pose "right." Then I realized that constant refining is the pose.

MODIFYING THE POSE

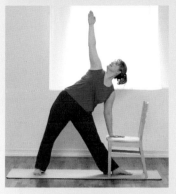

If balancing poses are a challenge, try this gentle modification: Position a chair with the seat facing your left leg. In Step 3 rest your left hand on the seat and straighten your right arm.

3 When you cannot reach forward with your left arm any more, rotate your arms, bringing your left arm down and your right arm up so that they are vertical. Open up the right shoulder and press the back of your torso and shoulders into an imaginary wall behind you. Remain here for 5 deep Ujjayi breaths. Reverse the steps and repeat on the other side.

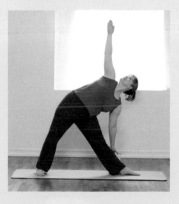

Practice Triangle with a block for a deeper stretch in the side of your waist. In 5-Pointed Star (inset, p78), position a block by the back edge of your left foot. In Step 3 rest your left hand on the block. Repeat on the other side.

EXTENDED TRIANGLE

Once you feel balanced in Triangle pose, add the lunge of the forward leg to enter
Extended Triangle. In this posture you will experience an even greater stretch of
the sides of your body. I believe that learning how to exit Extended Triangle is just
as important as holding the pose. Use the exhale in Step 3 to propel yourself up
without leaning heavily on your bent leg. Your breath will help you in every move.

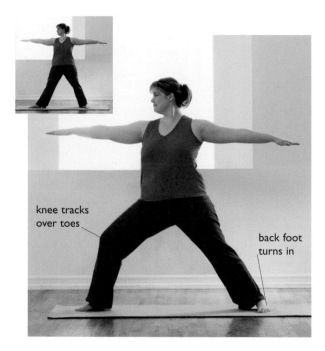

knee tracks
over toes

back foot
turns in

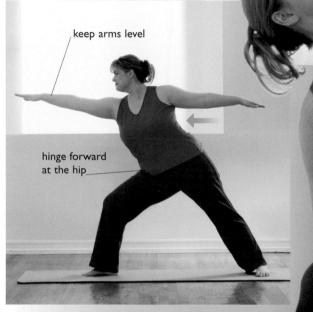

keep arms level

hinge forward
at the hip

1 Begin in 5-Pointed Star (inset). Inhaling,
turn your right foot out 90° as you gaze
at your outstretched fingertips. Come into
a lunge with your right leg. Breathe.

2 Exhaling, reach toward the front of your mat
through your right fingertips and hinge at
the hips. Imagine that your arms are resting on
a big table. Do not let them drop down toward
the floor. If they drop you have worked
beyond the strength of your abdominals.

Feeling the stretch is a lot more fun than striving to imitate your teacher, another student, or your idea of what the pose "should" look like.

MODIFYING THE POSE

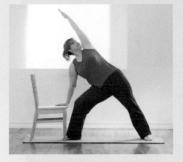

If balancing poses are a challenge, use this gentle modification of Extended Triangle: Position a chair at the front of your mat with the seat facing you. In Step 3 rest your left hand on the seat of the chair and straighten your right arm.

3 When you cannot slide forward with your right arm anymore, lower it and rest your forearm on your bent leg. Extend your left arm on a diagonal so that it forms a long line from your extended leg. As you breathe, rotate your left armpit up toward the sky. Take 5 deep Ujjayi breaths. Reverse the steps to exit the pose and repeat on the other side.

WATCH OUT FOR

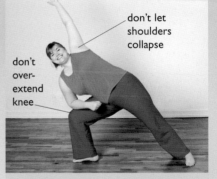

don't let shoulders collapse

don't over-extend knee

Be mindful to keep your knee at or behind your ankle. You should always be able to see your toes—otherwise you are overextending your knee.

HALF MOON

Turning sideways up the wall in Half Moon pose reminds me of that wild amusement park ride where centrifugal force flattens people into the walls of a spinning machine. In Half Moon, the wall provides you with a support and an important contact point for alignment—if you're peeling off of it, you are moving out of the pose. Half Moon improves hip flexibility, balance, and concentration as well as leg and abdominal strength. And it's really fun.

keep arms vertical

press shoulders into wall

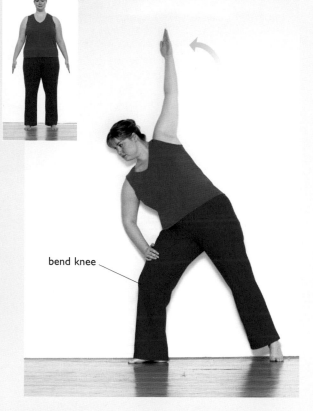

bend knee

press down through foot

1 Stand with your back to a wall (inset). Turn your right foot out 90° as you step your legs apart. Bend your right knee and draw your left leg back, sweeping your left arm up at the same time.

2 Exhale as you straighten your right leg and simultaneously lift your left leg until it is parallel with the floor. Keep your back pressed into the wall at all times.

3 Breathe deeply as you reach out through your left heel and press your back into the wall for support. Let your gaze travel up to your fingertips when you feel stable. Remember to keep your arms vertical. If you feel wobbly, look straight ahead. Remain here for 5–10 Ujjayi breaths. Reverse the steps to lower yourself with the support of the wall and repeat on the other side.

keep foot flexed

keep buttocks
pressed into wall

squeeze
thighs

MODIFYING THE POSE

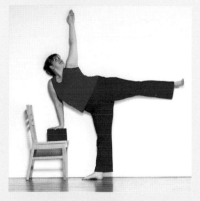

If you feel very wobbly in the pose, bring a chair to the wall with the seat facing you. As you go into the full pose in Step 3, rest your hand on the seat and push down strongly. Remember to keep pressing into the wall.

For more support, place a block or a couple of phone books on the seat of a chair to bring the surface closer to your hand. Now you don't need to bend over so far. Keep pressing into the wall for support.

FORWARD FOLD REST

This delightful inversion quiets the mind after the strong stimulation of the first Standing poses. Allow gravity to do the work for you as you visualize the space between your vertebrae expanding with each breath. I like to practice the modification resting my body on the back of a chair whenever my hamstrings are tight. If you have uncontrolled high blood pressure, detached retina, or glaucoma, avoid this pose.

MEGA TIP

Use the chair modification, below, if you have an "apple" body type and carry your weight in your belly. You can also use the modification if you have tight hamstrings.

slide buttocks up wall

let head hang

feet are one small step from the wall

MODIFYING THE POSE

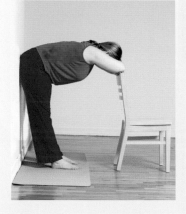

Place a chair in front of the mat with the back of the chair facing you. Rest your forearms and forehead on the back of the chair in order to reduce the degree of the forward fold.

1 Standing with your back against a wall (inset), exhale and slowly walk your feet one small step away from the wall. Inhale and then exhale as you peel your head, shoulders, and upper back off the wall and into a forward fold. Hold the pose, resting in it for 5–10 breaths. Then roll up slowly, pressing your back into the wall. Pause, standing upright, and breathe.

SHOULDER OPENER

A yoga strap (or a men's tie) is a great prop for opening the shoulder joint. Do a few rounds of Shoulder Opener with a very wide grip on the strap and then move your hands closer together, if you are able to. You'll know you are straining if your hands break away when you draw your arms up and back behind you. This move is a great preparation for Stargazer on the page that follows (see pp86-87).

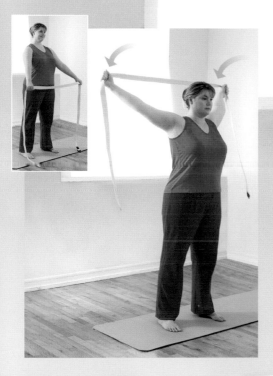

2 Exhale as you lower your hands all the way down to your buttocks. Keep the movement smooth and the strap taught. Don't jut your chin forward. To come out of the posture, inhale as you lift your arms back up and in front of you. Repeat 5 times.

1 Clasp a yoga strap or a men's tie in your hands, holding it taught. Keep your arms wider than shoulder-width apart. Make sure your wrists are straight, not flexed up or down (inset). Inhale as you sweep your arms overhead, keeping the strap taught. Widen the space between your hands if the stretch becomes too intense.

STARGAZER

Shoulder Opener (see p85) is a great way to warm up for the back bend in Stargazer. In this pose, when I backbend, I imagine my heart expanding, filling with divine inspiration. When you bend back, gently squeeze your buttocks to protect your lower back—Squeeze them before you start the back bend. Avoid bending your back if you've had a recent injury, and practice with caution if your balance is shaky.

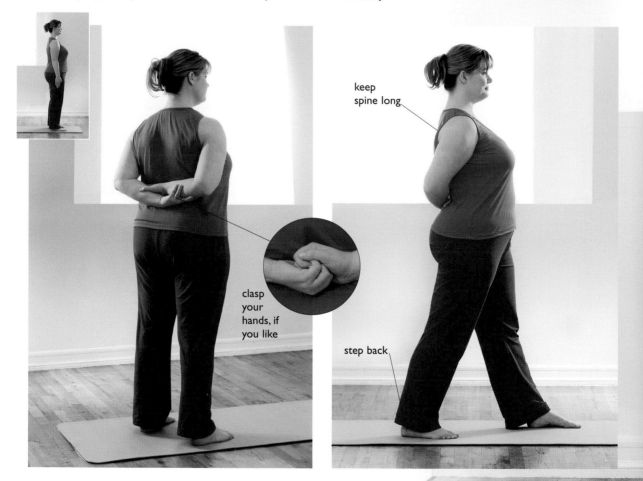

keep spine long

clasp your hands, if you like

step back

1 Begin in Mountain pose, with your arms at your sides (inset). Exhaling, bring your hands behind your back and clasp your forearms. Squeeze your shoulders back and down.

2 Inhale, then exhale, taking a small step back with your right foot. Keep your toes facing forward and your feet parallel, as if they were on two railroad tracks.

lift heart

enjoy the
belly stretch

arch back

3 Inhale, then exhale, as you lift your chest and arch back. Squeeze your buttocks to protect your lower back and take 5 deep Ujjayi breaths. Reverse steps and change sides.

lightly squeeze
buttocks

keep feet
parallel

EAGLE

In any balancing pose the more rigid you become—in an effort to stay upright—the more likely it is that you will fall out of the pose. Practicing Eagle develops the poise and concentration you need to stay balanced. Wrapping the arms in Eagle stretches the backs of your arms and shoulders. Squatting on one leg improves balance and strengthens the supporting leg.

> **CAUTION**
> Avoid hand wrapping in Eagle if you have:
> • carpal tunnel syndrome
> • a recent wrist injury or acute discomfort

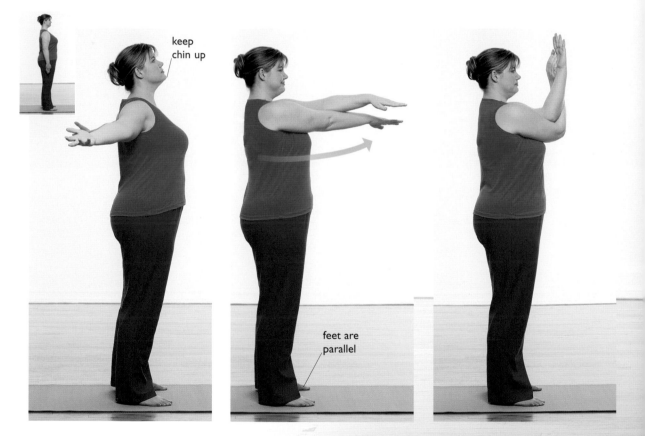

keep chin up

feet are parallel

1 Begin in Mountain pose, arms at your sides, feet parallel, thighs hugging muscle to bone (inset). Inhale. Slowly sweep your arms up and out behind you.

2 Exhale, as you bring your arms in front of you. Cross your arms at the elbows. Take a breath. Exhale, melting your shoulder blades back and down.

3 Inhale. Raise your forearms perpendicular to the mat. Exhale. Bind your hands one on top of the other. Keep your wrists perpendicular to the floor.

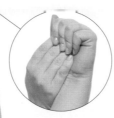

neatly curl the fingers of your left hand over the fingers of your right hand

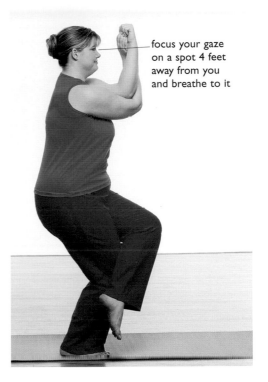

focus your gaze on a spot 4 feet away from you and breathe to it

4 Inhale, slowly shifting your weight to the right leg. Exhale and wrap your left leg over the standing leg. Press your inner thighs together to increase the wrap.

5 Inhale, then exhale, bending the supporting leg as you send your tailbone back and down. Take 5 deep Ujjayi breaths. Then stand up slowly and repeat on the other side.

keep weight on standing leg

MODIFYING THE POSE

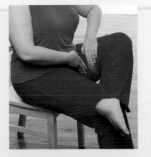

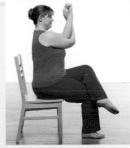

Using your fingertips, roll your inner thigh flesh up and out to create more space between your thighs for a deeper leg wrap.

Now take your hands away, press your thighs together, and wrap your forearms. Keep your spine long and straight.

AWKWARD POSE

Aren't yoga poses aptly named? The deep squat in Awkward pose makes me feel like I'm poised over a barbecue flame. Remember the rule about knee safety and be sure that you can see all your toes as you squat. Got knee pain? Awkward pose will rapidly strengthen your quadriceps (thigh muscles) and hamstrings so that you can better stabilize your knees going up and down stairs or simply sitting and standing.

keep back straight

2 Exhale as you sink down into an imaginary chair, pointing your tailbone behind you. Bring your weight onto your heels and off your toes. Keep your spine straight and your shoulder blades back and down. Hold the pose for 5–10 deep Ujjayi breaths.

put weight on heels, not toes

1 Begin in Mountain pose, feet parallel at a comfortable hip width. Inhale, sweeping your arms overhead. Keep your shoulders back and down.

arms reach up

Use Ujjayi breathing in this pose to focus and whittle away at all the negative voices that have ever made you feel that you can't measure up!

bend knees

MODIFYING THE POSE

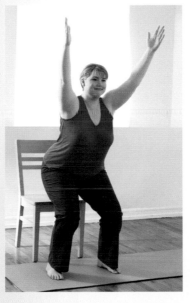

If you'd like a gentler alternative to the full pose in Step 2, sit at the edge of a chair. Inhale as you raise your arms overhead and lift yourself a few inches off the seat. Exhaling, sit right back down. Repeat 5–10 times to build leg strength in the pose. Sit back down when you need a rest.

INTENSIFYING THE POSE

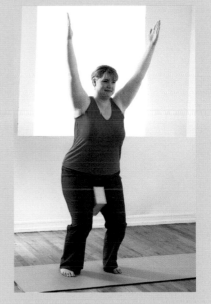

To strengthen the inner thighs, place a block between them and keep it there for the duration of the pose. Keep squeezing the block with your thighs to keep it from slipping out. See if you can roll the block forward a bit and then back again by rolling your inner thighs out and back in.

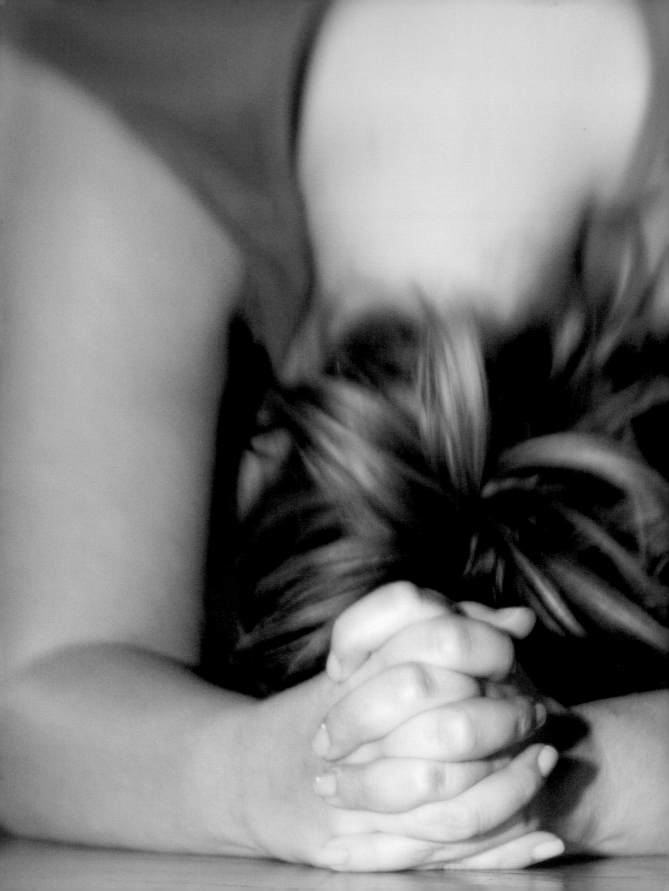

WALL POSES AND INVERSIONS

A wall—or even your front door—is a great partner for practicing yoga in Wall Poses and Inversions. When I first started practicing yoga, I had a lot of wrist soreness in Down Dog because I didn't know how to use my leg strength. Wall Flow teaches you how to engage your legs in Dog without putting weight on your wrists. Those of you who are ready for a thrill can try Handstand. It excites and inspires me! Why don't you start by building arm strength in Dolphin? You'll get to Handstand soon, trust me. This section ends with the bliss of Legs up the Wall and the rejuvenating Half Shoulder Stand.

WALL FLOW

Wall Flow is a moderately aerobic pose sequence that will get your blood pumping and stretch your legs and back. In this flow, you will be introduced to Half Dog (see Step 3 and Step 6), a moderate version of Down Dog pose. Wall Flow is my personal take on Sun Salute. Traditionally, this posture is a warm-up for standing poses. However, I've found that Sun Salute doesn't warm me up, because I constantly have to stop to "move the flesh" (see pp22–23) whenever I lunge. Other students, in classes I've taken, are ready for round two of the traditional pose, while I'm still on the floor! Wall Flow works for me because the upright placement of my torso means there is no flesh to move as I lunge.

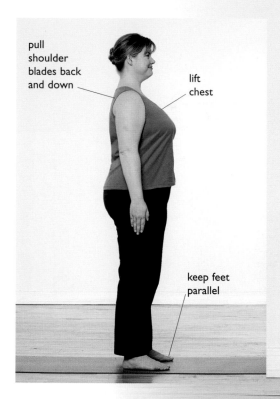

pull shoulder blades back and down

lift chest

keep feet parallel

2 Exhaling, lean forward and place your hands on the wall in front of you. Your hands should be shoulder-width apart with your fingers pointing up the wall and spread wide.

1 Begin in Mountain pose, hands at sides. Position your mat at a right angle to the wall. Stand a step or two from the wall.

press heels into floor

hands are
shoulder-width
apart

squeeze
abdominals

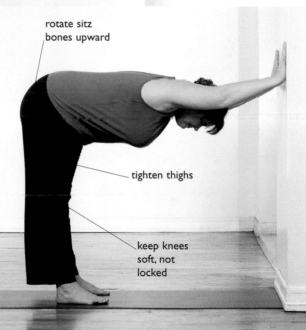

rotate sitz
bones upward

tighten thighs

keep knees
soft, not
locked

3 Inhale and then exhale, slowly sliding your hands
down the wall as you walk your feet back into
Half Dog. Take 5 deep Ujjayi breaths, feeling the strong
movement of your belly as you breathe. Contract your
thigh muscles to allow the backs of your legs to open.
Press back through your buttocks to lengthen your
spine while you keep your palms glued to the wall.

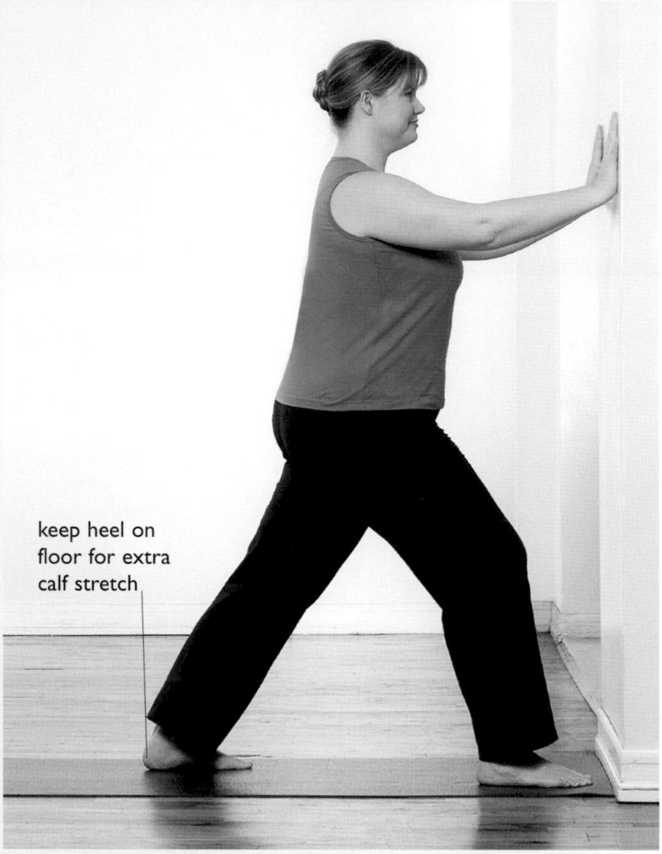

keep heel on
floor for extra
calf stretch

squeeze
shoulder
blades down

4 Inhale as you lunge your right foot
and simultaneously walk your hands
up the wall to straighten your torso.

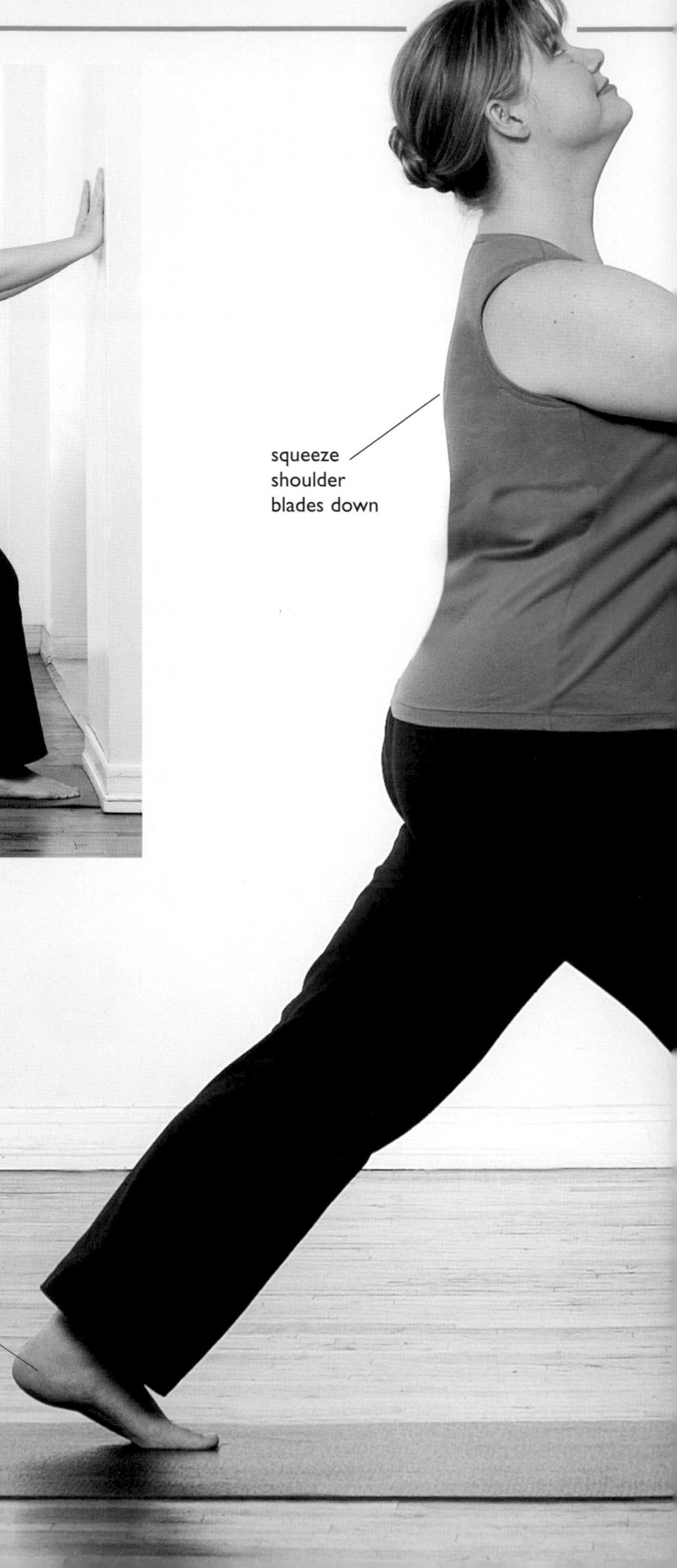

keep heel lifted
for a less intense
calf stretch

lift chest

Wall Flow is an excellent stretch for the back. It is particularly relaxing after several hours of sitting either at your desk or in a car.

press hands into wall

keep back flat

5 Exhale as you slide your hands up the wall, drawing your shoulder blades back and down. Press your palms into the wall as you lift your chest upward and gaze toward the sky for a gentle back bend. Breathe here for 5 deep Ujjayi breaths.

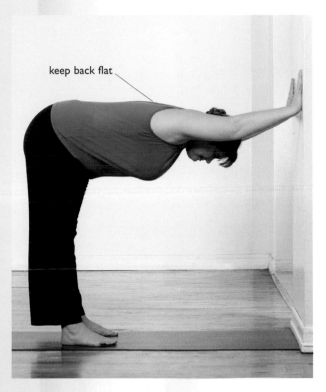

6 Exhale as you step your right foot back, sliding your hands down the wall to return to Half Dog. Keep your back flat as a table. Breathe here for 5 deep Ujjayi breaths. Repeat the lunge with your other leg and reverse the steps, returning to Mountain in Step 1. Repeat Wall Flow, alternating legs, until you break into a light sweat.

DOWN DOG

Down Dog is my absolute favorite yoga pose because it works the whole body while it calms the mind and spirit. In Down Dog you are balancing, standing, and inverting all at once. Start with Half Dog from Wall Flow (see p95) and when you feel confident in Half Dog, try Down Dog. Don't worry about keeping your heels on the floor at first. Instead, focus on taking the weight off your arms by working your thighs and lengthening your spine.

> ### CAUTION
> Avoid Down Dog if you have:
> • uncontrolled high blood pressure
> • detached retina or glaucoma
> • carpal tunnel syndrome
> • elbow soreness or ankle injury
> • hamstring injury

1 Start on your hands and knees. Take 5 deep Ujjayi breaths, observing the movement of your belly as you breathe. Make sure your hands are directly under your shoulders and your back is flat.

pedal feet in place on mat

2 Inhaling, lift your hips up into the air. Draw your thighs back toward the wall behind you and pedal your feet several times as you walk in place, breathing in and out.

BREAST BINDING

You may wish to bind your breasts for this inversion. For instructions see p23. First, try the posture without a strap, as I am doing in the photo below. If you can breathe freely, you don't need to bind.

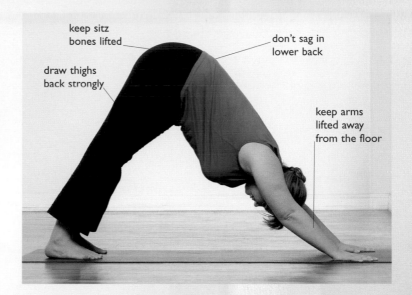

keep sitz bones lifted

don't sag in lower back

draw thighs back strongly

keep arms lifted away from the floor

3 Draw your thighs back strongly as your feet come to stillness in the full expression of Down Dog. It is more important to take the weight off your hands by learning to engage your legs than it is to keep your heels flat on the floor.

keep head in line with inner elbows

press down through base of knuckles

keep back of arms lifted

keep weight off wrists

MODIFYING THE POSE

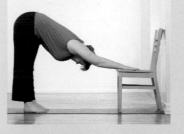

If you have tight hamstrings, place a chair against a wall, the seat facing you. Position your hands on the seat. This modifier is a very good transition from Half Dog (see Wall Flow, p95).

HANDSTAND

My first yoga teacher said that we would all do a handstand at the end of the semester. No excuses. I was so scared, my palms were sweating! On the fateful day when I kicked up the wall and was held aloft, I actually screamed as I balanced. It was amazing to be upside down—I'll always remember that feeling of terror and glee. Want to try it?

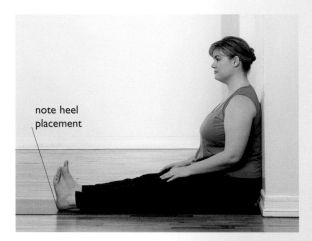

note heel placement

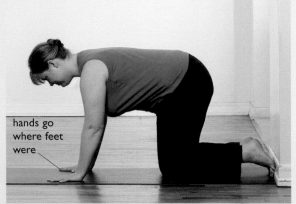

hands go where feet were

1 To place your hands correctly in Steps 2–4, sit with your back against a wall, your legs straight out. Note where your heels are on the mat: This is one leg length, and it is where you will place your hands when you invert in Step 4.

2 Get onto your hands and knees, keeping your hands shoulder-width apart. Place them exactly where your feet were in Step 1. Breathe, feeling the movement of your belly as you inhale and exhale.

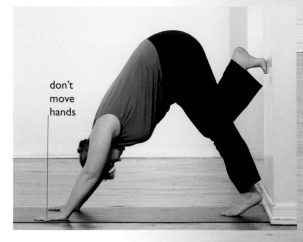

don't move hands

3 Inhaling, walk your right foot up the wall as you straighten your left leg and lift your buttocks. Place your right foot on the wall at the same level as your buttocks.

> **CAUTION**
>
> Avoid Handstand if you have:
> - high blood pressure
> - glaucoma or detached retina
> - inner ear infection
> - wrist, elbow, or shoulder sensitivity

4 Exhaling, press strongly into the wall with your right foot to straighten the right leg as you quickly lift your left foot up to join the right foot. Remain here and take 5 deep Ujjayi breaths. Use your exhales to really squeeze your abdominals and steady your torso.

press feet into wall

BREAST BINDING

You may wish to bind your breasts for this inversion (see instructions on p23). Try the pose without the strap, and note if your breasts impede your breathing. Not everyone will need it.

keep eyes open

don't lock elbows

DOLPHIN

Dolphin pose is the last vigorous inversion in this section. I teach Dolphin as a safe alternative to Handstand (see pp100-101) for plus-size students who want to experience the same sensations as the classic inversion—more blood to the brain, a quieting of the central nervous system, and a satisfying sense of calm. Because our weight would put too much stress on the delicate vertebrae of our necks—if we tried to balance on our heads— I and most of my students practice Dolphin instead.

elbows go directly under shoulders

CAUTION

Avoid Dolphin if you have:
• high blood pressure
• detached retina or glaucoma
• carpal tunnel syndrome
• elbow soreness

MEGA TIP

To avoid sinking down to the floor, keep your shoulders drawn down your back. In this inversion you may wish to bind your breasts. See p23 for instructions.

don't sink into shoulders

head skims surface of mat

1 Begin on your hands and knees, facing away from the wall (inset). Exhale as you lower your elbows directly under your shoulders, placing them on the mat exactly where your hands were (see inset). Rest your forearms on the floor and clasp your hands.

Turning upside down gives us a new perspective. Try it when you're stumped with a problem. See what happens.

INTENSIFYING THE POSE

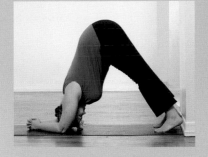

To increase the stretch, shorten the distance between your head and feet. This also provides a greater hamstring and calf stretch. Your head should just brush the top of the mat.

lower your heels

2 Inhale and exhale as you lift your hips toward the ceiling, straightening your legs and lowering your heels as close to the floor as possible. Breathe here for 5 deep Ujjayi breaths, allowing your head to brush the floor. Let gravity lengthen your neck.

LEGS UP THE WALL

Legs up the Wall relieves swelling and congestion in the legs and feet. In my job as a model I have to stand completely still for hours at a time while clothing designers drape and pin fabric on me. All that standing makes my feet throb by the end of the day. Fifteen minutes of Legs up the Wall has become my daily cocktail for leg health as soon as I get home from work.

> **MEGA TIP**
>
> Flexing and pointing your feet in Legs up the Wall helps drain retained fluid from your legs, a great tip from Dr. Jeff Migdow, holistic physician and Kripalu instructor.

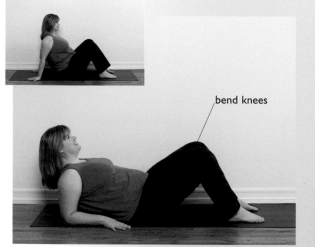

bend knees

1 Sit with your left side against a wall (inset). Exhaling, recline on your forearms, keeping your body flush against the wall.

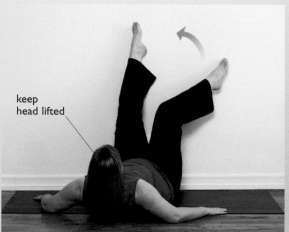

keep head lifted

2 Inhale and lift both legs, scooting your buttocks around as you turn your torso to face the wall. Keep your buttocks a few inches away from the wall.

3 On the exhale let your arms come out to a T position at shoulder height. Breathe here for at least 5 minutes—or as long as it feels comfortable for you.

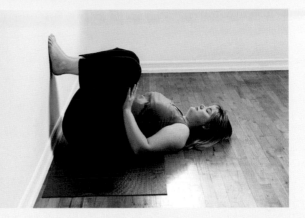

4 To exit the pose, slide your legs down the wall and bring your knees into your chest as you relax your lower back. Breathe here.

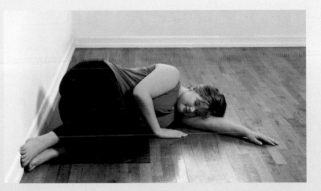

5 Roll to one side and relax in a fetal position, your head resting on your arm. Remain here for 5 deep breaths as you feel the effects of the pose.

HALF SHOULDER STAND

Half Shoulder Stand stimulates the thyroid, which is located at the base of the throat and regulates metabolism. This gentle inversion also promotes drainage of excess fluid in the legs and feet. Half Shoulder Stand quiets the mind, since the head is below the heart. Because you will be supporting your body weight on your shoulders in this pose, you may find it more comfortable to fold a thick yoga mat or a blanket under your upper back.

> ## CAUTION
> Avoid this pose if you have:
> - high blood pressure
> - sinusitis or head cold
> - neck injury or sensitivity
> - shoulder injury or sensitivity
> - inner-ear infection

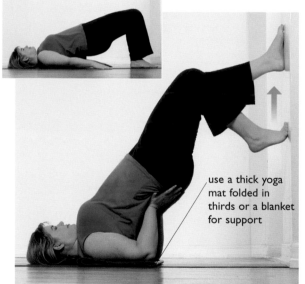

use a thick yoga mat folded in thirds or a blanket for support

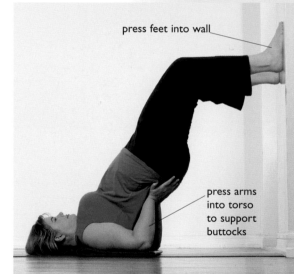

press feet into wall

press arms into torso to support buttocks

1 Begin on your back, knees bent, arms to your sides (inset). Supporting your buttocks with your hands, swing your left leg up and place your foot flat on the wall, pressing into it. Bring your right leg up next and press both feet into the wall.

2 Find a comfortable height for your feet. Press your feet into the wall. Squeeze your arms into the sides of your torso to provide good support for your buttocks. Breathe here for 5 deep breaths. Keep your head still and close your eyes if you like.

Once I've settled into a comfortable working stance I like to imagine that I'm melting away like a snowman on a sunny day.

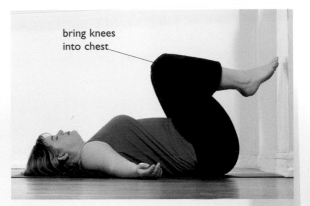

bring knees into chest

keep legs straight

4 To exit the pose walk your feet back down the wall and bring your knees into your chest as you exhale. Remain here for 5 deep breaths as you feel the effects of the pose.

support buttocks with hands

3 To come into the full expression of the pose, take your legs away from the wall and straighten them. Keep supporting your buttocks with your hands.

BREAST BINDING

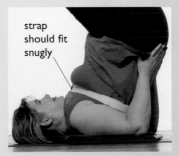

strap should fit snugly

Some of my students like to practice this pose with bound breasts because a strap keeps their chest from covering their mouth and inhibiting their ability to breathe. For instructions on how to use the strap see p23.

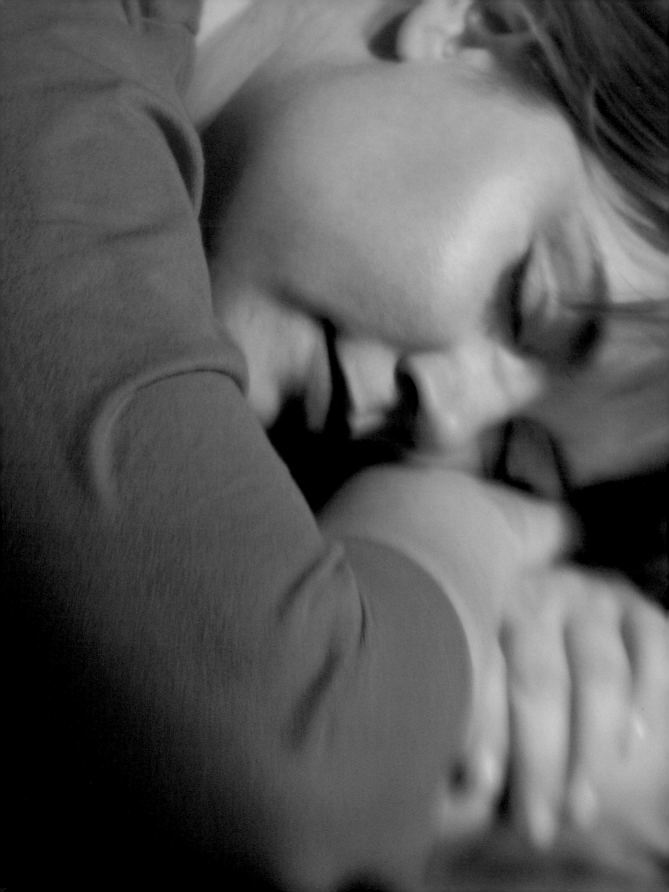

CLEANSING POSES

Cleansing poses work with the digestive and metabolic systems of the body. Fish pose, for example, stimulates the thyroid gland at the base of the throat, a natural treatment for a sluggish metabolism. Other Cleansing poses, such as Wind Reliever, Reclining Leg Stretch, and Reclining Tree, stimulate the abdominal region with either gentle pressure from the thighs or twisting action. These poses aid the process of digestion and are a great relief if you suffer from irritable bowel syndrome, gas, or constipation. Practice Cleansing poses sequentially to work with the natural cleansing systems of your body.

FISH

Fish pose stretches the front of the throat and the entire chest. When I practice this pose, my mouth opens slightly as my head arches backward. This is the only yoga pose where I advocate mouth breathing because it has a tendency to dry out the throat and tongue. The most important part of the pose is the entry and exit. *Always* keep your head in contact with the floor to protect your neck. If you feel any discomfort, come back down to the mat. Done correctly, Dirgha breathing (see pp26-27) in Fish looks like a wave rolling up and down your body.

> **MEGA TIP**
>
> I tell my students to slide onto the "yarmulke" at the back of their heads (not the crown of their heads) to safely exit the pose. Treat your neck gently!

1 Lie flat on your back, hands hugging your sides. Exhaling, flex your feet and squeeze your leg muscles as you breathe. Allow your eyes to close as you focus on breathing.

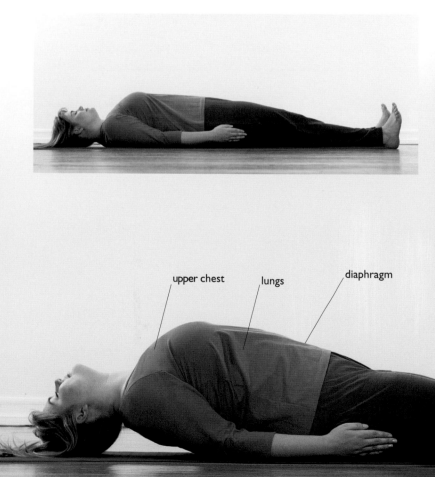

upper chest   lungs   diaphragm

2 Inhale, then exhale, and *without lifting your head off the floor* (this is most important for neck safety) slowly slide onto the back of your head. Take 5–10 deep Dirgha breaths, breathing first from your diaphragm, then from your lungs, and finally from your upper chest. Then release and rest.

RECLINING LEG CIRCLES

These leg circles allow you to explore the openness of your hips and the relative flexibility of your hamstrings. Be sure to keep your buttocks engaged and your exhales strong as you circle your legs. Notice if it is easier for you to open your leg out to the side or if you find it more comfortable to cross it over your body.

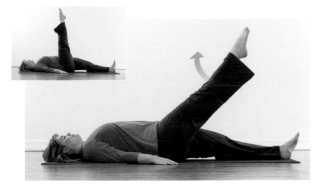

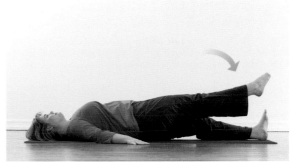

1 Lie flat on your back, inhale, and raise your right leg perpendicular to the floor (inset). Exhale and begin to draw a circle in the air with your leg.

2 As you circle the air with your leg, keep your upper body glued to the floor. Keep the nonworking leg engaged, foot flexed.

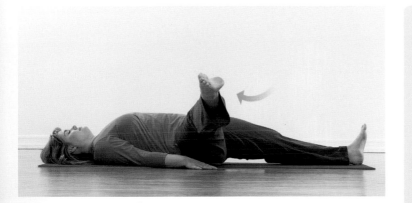

MODIFYING THE POSE

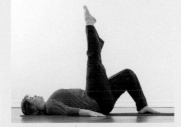

3 After you've completed a full circle going in one direction, go the other way. Repeat the circles as often as you like. Switch sides and circle in both directions with your other leg.

If you have a sore or weak lower back, try bending one of your knees to maintain the natural curve in your lower back. Keep the foot of your bent leg glued to the floor. Keep your circles small.

BRIDGE

Bridge pose is a great remedy for a weak or achy lower back because it strengthens the buttocks, hamstrings, and back erector muscles. The entry into Bridge gives you time to flex each vertebra, beginning at the tip of your tailbone and progressing gradually up to your shoulders. If I've been carrying a really heavy purse all day, practicing Bridge gives me a little chiropractic release between the shoulder blades as my weight presses into my upper back.

> **MEGA TIP**
> The tuck of the tailbone in Bridge is the same tuck as in Cat Tilt (see p50). Tucking the tailbone helps to create space between the vertebrae of your lumbar spine.

keep knees one
fist-width apart

1 Lie on your back. Inhaling, bring your feet in toward your buttocks, feet flat on the floor. Place your hands on the floor, palms down, fingertips reaching toward your heels.

After I hurt my lower back, Bridge was an integral part of my therapy. If you have lower back pain or weakness, try Bridge—it really helps.

INTENSIFYING THE POSE

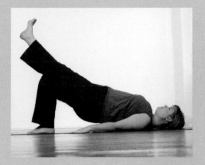

To challenge yourself, lift one leg while the other remains bent. Keep the lifted leg straight, then lift your hips to a comfortable height. As you hold the pose, concentrate on keeping your hips level. The hip of the straight leg has a tendency to dip down. Resist this!

keep hips lifted and tailbone tucked up

2 Exhaling, curl your tailbone up as you squeeze your buttocks and press your feet and arms strongly into the floor. Keep your buttocks lifted for 5–10 deep breaths. Exhale, and slowly lower them to the floor.

press the backs of your arms into the floor

HAPPY BABY

As you open your hips and inner thighs in Happy Baby pose, try to imagine that your joints are still soft and flexible like those of a little child. Do not press your lower back into the mat or overarch in an attempt to grab your feet. You may not come anywhere near them right away! That's OK—just grab your pants legs and hang on to them as you let your inner thighs relax and release as you breathe.

> **MEGA TIP**
>
> It's more important to focus on letting your knees melt down toward your armpits than to reach your feet. You can hold your pants legs, too.

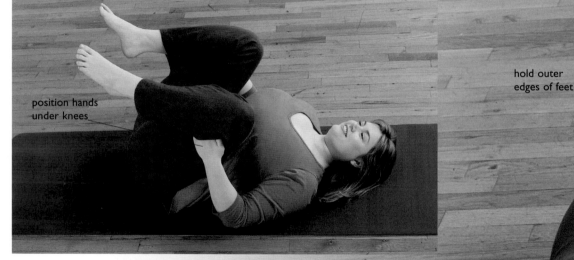

position hands under knees

hold outer edges of feet

1 Lie on your back, feet flat on the foor. Slowly exhale as you draw one leg and then the other toward your body. Position your hands under your knees in order to draw your legs toward you. If you have an abundant belly, take a moment to smooth it up and out of your hip crease.

flex toes toward
your nose for an
extra calf stretch

The reclining stretch in Happy
Baby works the skill of patience.
As you breathe, you must surrender
to the unfolding of your inner
thigh. You can't rush the stretch.
It unfolds in its own time.

2 Lift the soles of your feet up as if you were
going to stand on the ceiling—shins vertical.
Clasp the outside edges of your feet. If you
cannot reach your feet, hold onto your ankles,
calves, or pants legs. Breathe here for 5–10
breaths, then lower and relax.

RECLINING LEG STRETCH

This classic stretch enables you to feel your hamstrings and calf muscles unwind and lengthen. Reclining Leg Stretch is one of the training complements to Down Dog (see pp98–99). You can't begin to take weight into your legs without the dual action of leg strength plus hamstring flexibility. Use a yoga strap looped around the bottom of your foot in order to reach your foot without lifting your shoulders off the mat. All parts of your body should relax, except for the working leg.

> **MEGA TIP**
>
> If you don't have a yoga strap, you can use a bathrobe or coat tie instead, but make sure it is at least as long as your leg so that you don't have to strain to reach the ends.

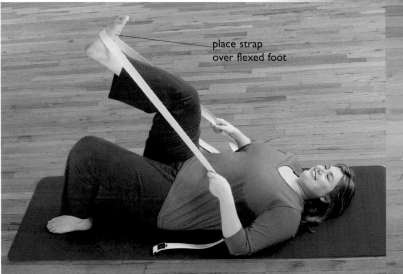

place strap over flexed foot

keep foot flat

2 Exhaling, slowly press your flexed foot straight up toward the ceiling. Keep the backs of your arms flat on the floor and your shoulders down. Reach up strongly through your heel in order to stretch your hamstrings.

1 Begin by lying on your back on the floor, your legs bent and feet flat. Place a flexed foot into a yoga strap, holding on to the ends of the strap with your hands. Rest the backs of your arms on the floor and relax your upper body.

press foot up

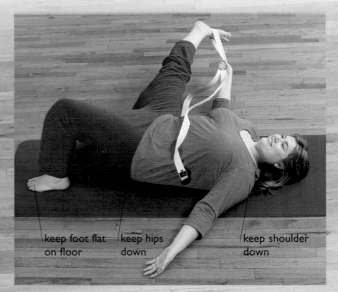

keep foot flat | keep hips | keep shoulder
on floor | down | down

3 Ater 5–10 deep breaths, slowly exhale your right leg out to the side, holding the strap in your right hand. Let your left arm relax and drop out to the side. Keep the foot of your bent leg flat on the floor. After 5–10 deep breaths, inhale and bring your leg back up to center. Slowly lower it to the floor, then repeat the leg stretch on the other side.

RECLINING TREE

Tree pose, as it is practiced on the floor, involves exactly the same principles as the standing version of Tree (see pp76–77). As you draw your foot up your nonworking leg, there is a tendency for your hip to follow, bringing your hips out of alignment. Keep your hips level. This will provide a gentle release in your lower back. Rest here and let gravity do the job of opening up your inner thighs. Stay as long as you need to in order to feel the release.

> **MEGA TIP**
>
> As you enter the pose in Step 2, work both hips down evenly. You may even wish to press your hipbones with your fingertips to encourage them to melt down.

keep foot flexed

1 Begin by lying on your back, knees bent, feet flat on the floor. Slowly extend one leg, keeping it long and flexing the extended foot.

Does Reclining Tree seem familiar? Its sister is your habitual "good morning" stretch in bed, arms overhead. Let out a yawn or a sigh and let go.

place foot against side of knee or inner thigh

2 Inhale and exhale as you drop the bent leg out to the side and place your foot flat against your inner thigh. Remain here for 5 deep breaths.

3 Inhale and sweep your arms overhead, squeezing your shoulder blades down your back. Remain here for 5 deep breaths. Release and repeat on the other side.

keep hips level

WIND RELIEVER

Wind Reliever is a natural aid to digestion and the source of much amusement and embarrassment for my yoga students because it really works! The three-part sequence of squeezes in this pose follow the natural progression of digestion. First, squeeze the ascending colon on the right side of your body; then squeeze the transverse colon that runs across your belly. Finally, squeeze the descending colon on the left side of your body. An abundant belly is a an advantage in this pose because it gives you more substance to press on your organs!

MEGA TIP

If you have a sore or weak lower back, bring only one leg at a time up to your body. Don't bring both legs up at the same time. In Steps 1 and 3 leave one of your legs bent, foot flat on the floor.

keep feet relaxed

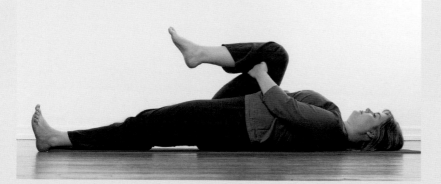

1 Exhaling, bend your right leg, hugging it into your body with both hands and clasping the back of your right thigh. On each exhale, squeeze the right leg into your body. Breathe deeply as you inhale and exhale for 5 breath cycles.

2 Inhale and draw both legs up to your body, hands clasping the backs of both thighs. On each exhale squeeze both legs into your body. Breathe deeply as you inhale and exhale for 5 breath cycles.

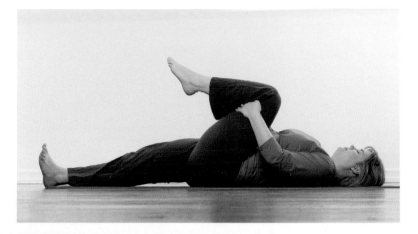

3 Inhaling, extend your right leg along the floor. Keep your left leg bent and drawn into your chest. On each exhale squeeze the left leg into your body. Breathe deeply as you inhale and exhale for 5 breath cycles. To come out of the pose, lower your left leg to the floor.

hug legs into body

keep forehead level with chin to prevent overarching neck

KNEE DOWN TWIST

Knee Down Twist provides a gentle stretch for the back while opening up the shoulder joint. Aim to keep the back of your arms glued to the floor as best as you can, as you flop your knees over to one side. Your shoulder will pop up away from the floor as you come all the way over. That's natural. Imagine that you're melting your armpit back down into the floor and feel the shoulder joint opening. Notice where you feel the most sensation in the twist. Breathe deeply into that place with the intention of spreading the stretch out and up and down the length of your spine.

MEGA TIP

For an added stretch, turn your head and look back in the opposite direction from your knees. If this is too much, you can look in the direction that you are twisting for less stretch.

place a small pillow between your legs for additional support if needed

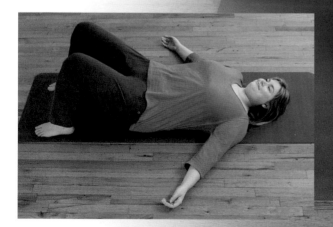

1 Begin by lying comfortably on a mat, your legs extended. Exhaling, bring your feet toward your buttocks and rest them flat on the floor.

2 Inhale your arms up to T position at shoulder height. Exhale and drop your knees to the right side, allowing your left hip to lift into the air. Breathe here for 5 deep breaths. Inhale up to center, keeping your arms pressed down. Then exhale over to the left side for 5 breaths.

Knee Down Twist, like Wind Reliever,
is a natural aid for constipation or gas.
Do it on an empty stomach—not after
a big Thanksgiving dinner.

relax hands

keep shoulders
relaxed on the floor

INTENSIFYING THE POSE

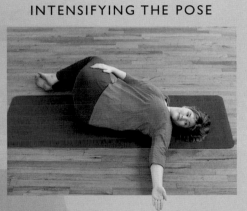

To deepen the twist in this pose, place
your right hand on top of your raised left
hip and then gently pull the hip toward
you as you breathe for several rounds.

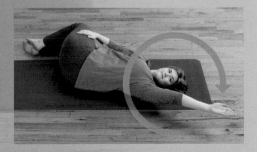

As you breathe in Step 2, make big circles
around your body with your outstretched
arm. Reach through your fingertips and focus
on making contact with either the floor, the
mat, or your body, as you explore the space
around you for several rounds.

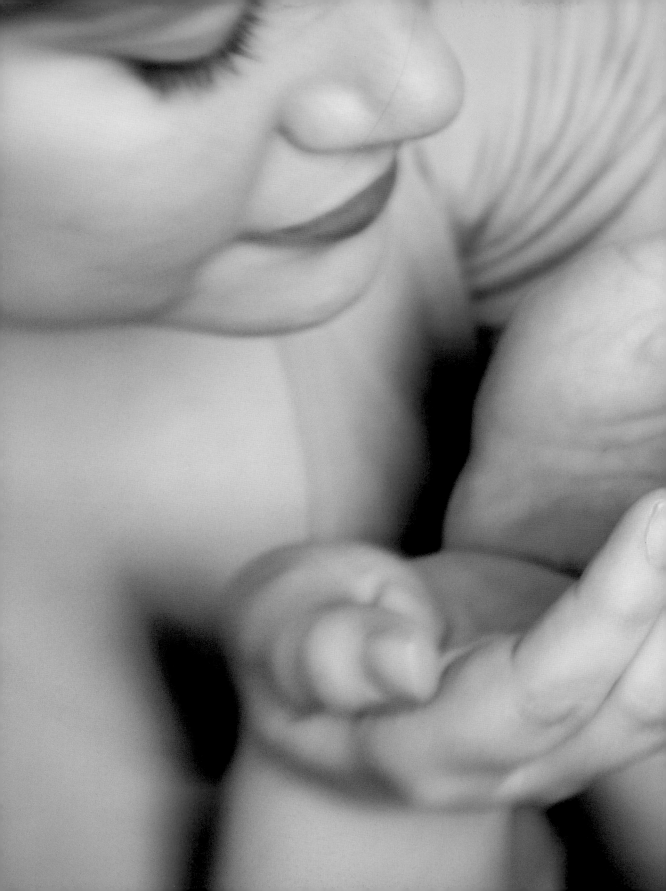

QUIET POSES

After you have warmed, worked, and stretched your body, you are primed to enter Quiet Poses. Belly-down poses such as Windshield Wiper Legs and Boat heighten your body awareness, helping you to judge—from the inside out—if you are in correct alignment. All Quiet Poses work with the skill of introversion: The body is quiet and the mind quiets, too. When this happens, you naturally fall silent in Corpse and begin to let go of deep tensions. Ending your practice with Meditation seals the experience of peaceful silence.

CROCODILE

Crocodile pose (and chocolate) is my answer to PMS-y days. Lying on your belly is a primal way to affirm safety. When animals curl up into a protective stance in the wild, they always cover their bellies. Give your belly the support of the floor and imagine that you are letting all the organs in your body melt downward. Feel your back lift and lower as you take your breath into the sides of your waist and the back of your body.

> **MEGA TIP**
>
> If you have a sore lower back, rest your pelvis on a pillow or folded blanket in Crocodile, and take your time entering and exiting the pose.

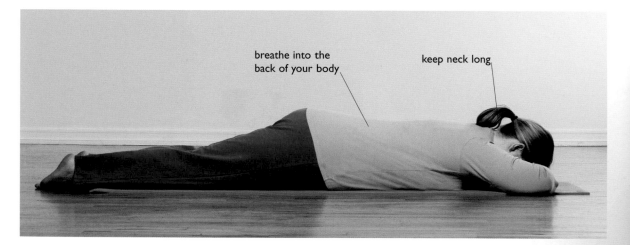

breathe into the back of your body

keep neck long

1 Lie on your belly. Move the flesh of your abdomen toward your head, so that you can feel your hipbones make contact with the floor. Smooth your breasts down, away from your neck and out to the sides. Bring your big toes together and let the outside edges of your feet fall to the sides. Fold your arms under your forehead and close your eyes. Breathe here for 10 deep breaths.

After you shed the layers of physical tension, sleep deprivation, and resistance, you will arrive at a very quiet place inside yourself—returning to your source.

WINDSHIELD WIPER LEGS

Windshield Wiper Legs is an instinctual yoga pose. I never have to give my students the instructions twice. If you want immediate relief from lower back tension, this is the pose for you. If you have a friend or loved one who wants to support you in your practice, ask them to rub their hands together and then place those warm hands on your lower back as you practice. It feels great! Be sure to return the favor.

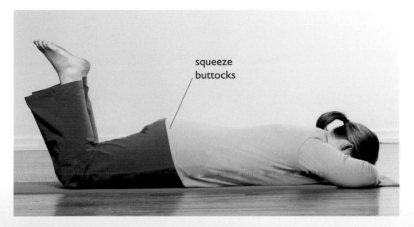

squeeze
buttocks

Try circling your legs like an eggbeater. Little kids love this move. I call it "crazy legs."

1 Lie on your belly in Crocodile (see opposite page). Inhale as you bend your knees, bringing your feet toward the ceiling.

2 Exhale as you drop your legs to the right. Inhale them up to center and then exhale them over to the left. Repeat 10 times or until you feel your lower back release all tension.

PIGEON

Pigeon pose provides a deep hip opening for the forward leg and a quad stretch for the back leg. Begin with your forward hip propped up on a pillow and then take the pillow away as you gain flexibility. If you feel any discomfort, pad the back knee or back ankle with a folded blanket. My students are partial to the Sleeping Pigeon variation in Step 4 because the forward fold also has a calming effect.

> **MEGA TIP**
>
> If you are experiencing knee discomfort, curl your back toes under, and straighten your back leg to keep your knee lifted off the floor in every step of the pose.

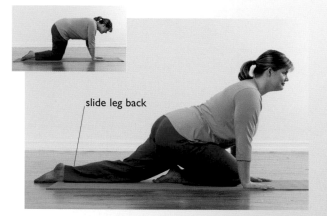

slide leg back

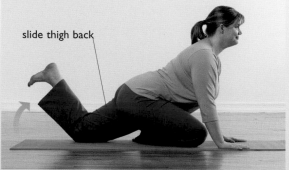

slide thigh back

1 Begin on your hands and knees (inset). Exhaling, slide your right knee forward between your hands as you slide your left leg behind you. Your right foot should be underneath your pubic bone.

2 Lift your left foot into the air and vigorously slide your left thigh back so that your weight rests on the top of your thigh rather than on your kneecap.

Relaxing in Sleeping
Pigeon, the practitioner
resembles a roosting
bird, her head tucked
under her wings,
preparing for nightfall.

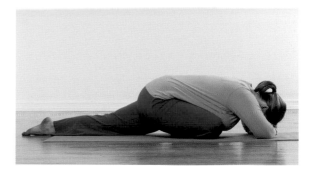

4 Exhaling, fold forward over your bent right leg
and come into Sleeping Pigeon. Make a pillow for
your head, either by folding your arms or stacking
one fist on top of the other. Stay here for 5–10 deep
Ujjayi breaths, then reverse the steps to return to the
start position. Repeat the pose with the other leg.

3 Inhaling, press
away from the
floor as you lift
your chest to
come into
Pigeon Pose.

lift chest forward

MODIFYING THE POSE

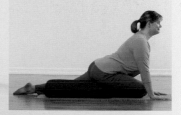

If your hips fall out of alignment
in Step 1, place a cushion or two
beneath your right hip as you slide
your right leg forward between your
hands. This will prevent you from
rolling dramatically to the right side.

LOCUST

If I say "Lift your right foot," do you automatically look at your right foot and then lift it? Yoga teaches us to sense where we are from the inside out. In Locust, you can't see the leg you are working, so you must trust your body wisdom to align yourself without visual assistance. Work through the pose step by step, using your senses to guide you. When you position yourself in Locust, don't forget to smooth the flesh of your abdomen away from your hipbones in order to breathe freely and feel your pelvis make contact with the floor.

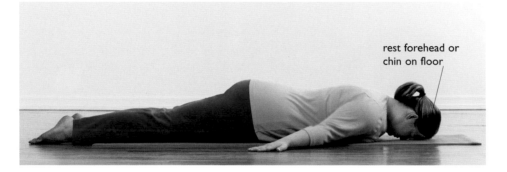

rest forehead or chin on floor

1 Lie down on your belly. Inhale and sweep your arms down to the sides of your waist, palms turned down and fingertips reaching toward your feet. Rest either your chin or your forehead on the floor, depending on your neck flexibility. Separate your feet hip-width apart and point your toes behind you.

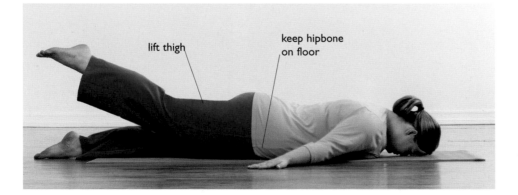

lift thigh

keep hipbone on floor

2 Exhale as you press your pubic bone into the floor and raise your right thigh straight up. It is more important to lift up through the thigh than the foot. Vigorously press both hipbones into the mat. Remain here for 5 deep breaths, then lower your leg and repeat on the other side.

BOAT

Boat pose works the entire back while providing a massage for the abdominal organs as your body rides waves of breath. When I first started practicing the pose I reached back so strongly through my arms and legs that my triceps and hamstrings were sore the next day. After some time, I noticed that my buttocks got sore from from overusing them in order to protect my lower back. As these sensations moved from part to part I knew my body was learning the pose. What do you feel when you practice?

rest forehead or chin on floor

1 Lie down on your belly. Smooth the flesh of your abdomen away from your hipbones. Reach back strongly through your fingers and toes, palms turned down.

2 Inhale. Feel your belly press into the floor as it expands. Exhaling, lift your arms, chest, head, and legs. Gaze straight ahead, not up, to avoid straining the back of your neck. Remain here for 5–10 deep breaths as your boat rides the waves of breath. Enjoy the sensation of bobbing up and down as you inhale and exhale.

keep neck long

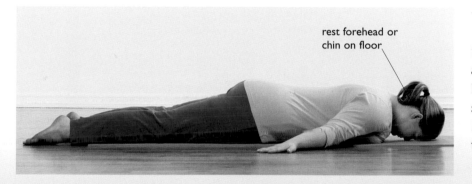

SPHINX

Sphinx pose is a gentle back bend that stretches the spine. Concentrate on keeping your neck long and your shoulder blades moving down your back so that you can puff your chest forward between your hands. If you are practicing with good form you will also feel your belly stretching all the way down to your pelvis. Sphinx relieves deep-seated tension in the abdomen, an area that many women feel they should "hold in" because it makes them look slimmer.

> **MEGA TIP**
> Be careful not to tilt your head too far back in Step 2 or you might compress the disks in your spine. A good way to avoid this is to gaze straight ahead, rather than up.

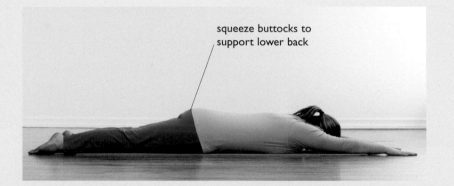

squeeze buttocks to support lower back

1 Lie on your belly. Inhaling, sweep your arms overhead, your palms reaching down through your fingertips. Exhaling, press your pubic bone down. Slide your elbows in toward your body one at a time. Stop when they are directly below your shoulders.

Although it doesn't look like much is happening in Sphinx, your entire spine is receiving a big stretch. Postures don't have to look dramatic to have dramatic results.

2 Roll your shoulders back and down as you draw your heart forward between your hands by pressing your palms back and down. Keep your head level to avoid straining your neck. Remain here for 5 deep breaths. Then lower your torso.

lift chest

press down
into forearms
for balance

CORPSE

Most of us find contemplation of death to be morbid and scary. In fact, when I first started teaching, I called Corpse pose "Deep Relaxation" because it sounded so much more pleasant than "Corpse." But I was avoiding the true meaning of the pose. In death, all of our wishing and striving is over. A corpse cannot act—surrender naturally occurs as we leave our earthly body behind. Corpse pose shows us the challenge and freedom of surrender: Lay down flat on your back. Let your feet and hands, palms facing up, fall out to the side. Breathe naturally, close your eyes, and allow the weight of your body to melt into the floor. Concentrate on relaxing every part of your body, staying awake and observant as you surrender to gravity.

> **MEGA TIP**
> Come out of Corpse twice as slowly as you think you need to: Roll onto your side and rest for several breaths in a fetal position. You are still in the pose, even though you are on the way out of it.

Slowly exiting from Corpse pose will preserve the experience of utter stillness, and the peacefulness will linger for hours after your practice.

MODIFYING THE POSE

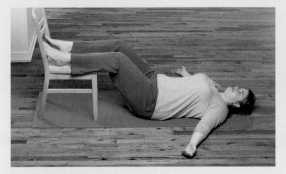

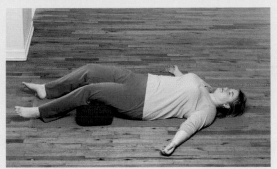

When I injured my lower back, I started Corpse pose with my legs resting on a kitchen chair and gradually lowered them to a cushion. Once you feel comfortable, allow each of your breaths to calm your mind and take you deeper into relaxation.

Place a firm pillow under your knees to ease lower back pain. It may also feel nice to place a slim book under your head or neck for more support. Some practitioners enjoy covering their eyes with a yoga tie or a small towel to deepen the mood of relaxation.

Imagine yourself sinking into warm sand as you let go and surrender to stillness.

MEDITATION

Begin in a seated posture (see photo, right, and caption). Before you meditate, practice several repetitions of Alternate Nostril breathing (see p29) until your breath slows naturally. Let your eyes close softly. If you find this makes you very sleepy, keep your eyes open and focus on the floor several feet in front of you. Breathe in. Feel the temperature of the air at the tip of your nostrils. As you breathe in, the air is cool. As you exhale, the air is warm from its passage through your body. Breathe this way, noting the difference in temperature at the tips of your nostrils with each inhale and exhale. Practice meditating like this for several minutes at the end of every yoga session.

MEGA TIP

As soon as you are aware that your thoughts have drifted, notice whether or not you are inhaling or exhaling. This will quiet your mind and give you a focal point for meditation.

The purpose of meditation is not to empty your mind of all thoughts—rather, it is meant to strengthen your ability to concentrate so that you can experience more of the present moment.

Sit with your back straight and settle your hands in your lap. Let your dominant hand be cradled by your nondominant hand. Allow your thumbs to kiss and your hands to be soft and relaxed. Breathe slowly.

MODIFYING THE POSE

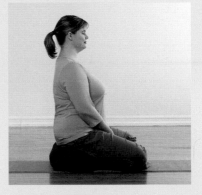

You can sit on a firm pillow or several folded blankets to elevate your hips and allow your spine to lengthen as you meditate. Let your breathing quiet your mind.

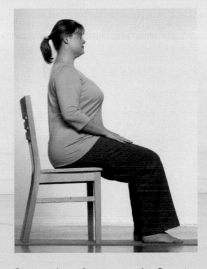

Sit in a chair, if sitting on the floor is uncomfortable for you. Remember to keep your spine long and your head up as you concentrate on slowing your breath. Let it relax you.

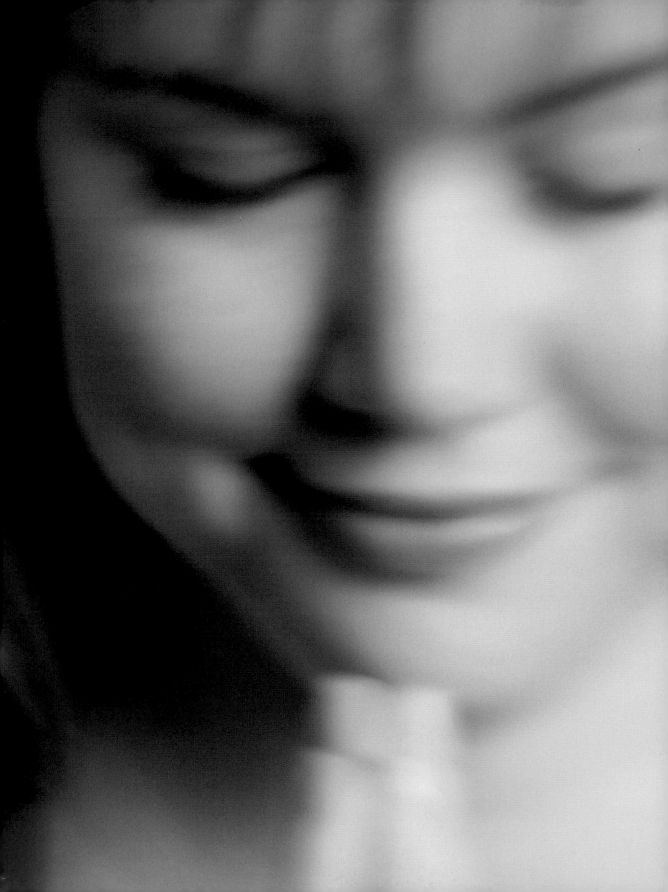

MEGAYOGA™ PROGRAMS

The 30-Minute Program, 60-Minute Program, and 90-Minute Program are meant for your lifelong development as a yoga practitioner. If you are a beginner, start with the 30-Minute Program for the first 6 months of your yoga practice. After you feel confident in all the poses of the 30-Minute Program, move on to the 60-Minute Program for months 6–18. The 90-Minute Program will grow with you from months 18 and beyond. Always start with Warm-Ups, even if you choose to practice your own sequence of poses. Pace yourself and remember that you are your own best teacher.

30-MINUTE PROGRAM

Start with the 30-Minute Program for the first 6 months of your yoga practice. This program teaches you basic breathing and strength-building skills. If you'd like to use any modifications, refer to the Modifying the Pose box for each pose. When you're ready for a challenge try the intensifiers. Don't forget to start your daily practice with centering (see p18) before warming up with the 30-Minute Program. End your practice with several minutes of meditation (see pp136–137).

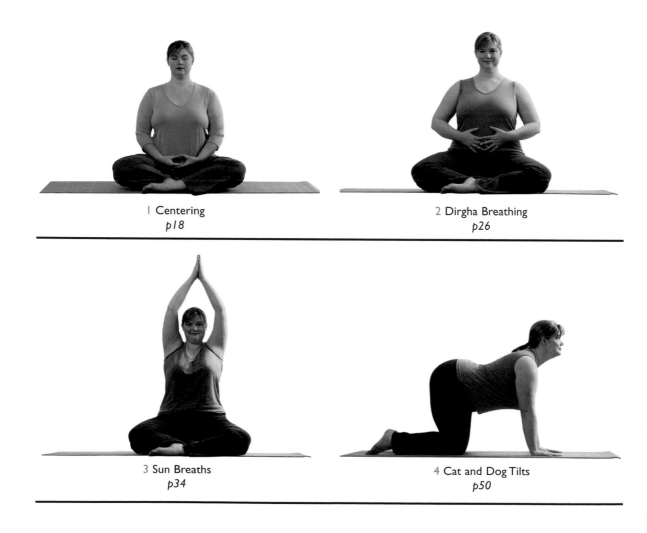

1 Centering
p18

2 Dirgha Breathing
p26

3 Sun Breaths
p34

4 Cat and Dog Tilts
p50

Commit to practicing the 30-Minute Program several days a week at a regular time. Carve out space for yourself to make practice a habitual part of your day.

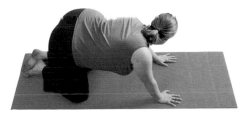

5 Kidney Squeeze
p53

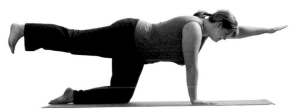

6 Table Balance
p52

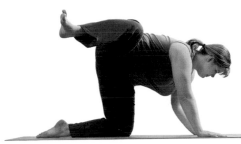

7 Fire Hydrants
p54

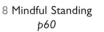

8 Mindful Standing
p60

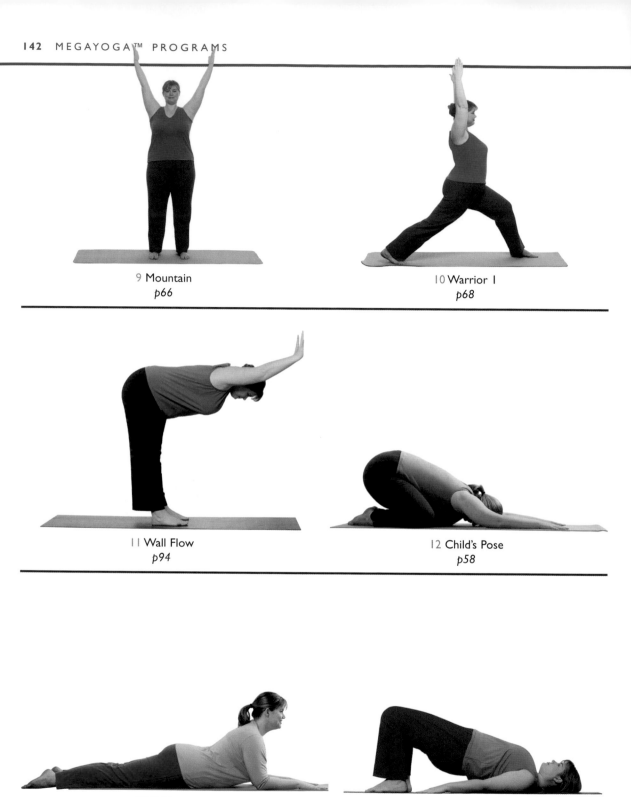

9 Mountain
p66

10 Warrior 1
p68

11 Wall Flow
p94

12 Child's Pose
p58

13 Sphinx
p132

14 Bridge
p112

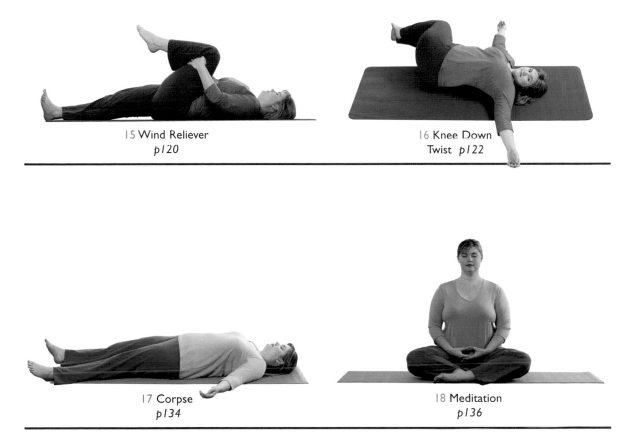

15 Wind Reliever
p120

16 Knee Down
Twist *p122*

17 Corpse
p134

18 Meditation
p136

Study the pictures of the poses,
note which ones require props,
and then assemble them—before
you begin your practice.

60-MINUTE PROGRAM

Move on to the 60-Minute Program for months 6–18 of your yoga practice. In this program you will work with poses that cultivate moving the flesh and breast-binding skills. These tools will prepare you to enter any yoga class at a gym or studio and adapt the poses to fit your body. You will get more enjoyment out of the class and maybe even teach your teacher about plus-size bodies so that she can help others! Be mindful to begin your practice with centering (see p18) before you warm up. And, of course, always end with several minutes of meditation (see pp136–137).

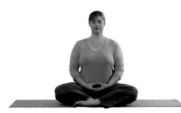

1 Centering
p18

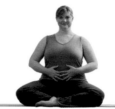

2 Dirgha Breathing
p26

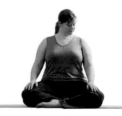

3 Neck Stretches
p32

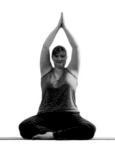

4 Sun Breaths
p34

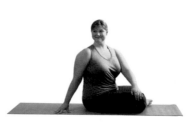

5 Seated Twist
p36

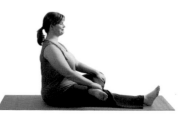

6 Ankle Rolls and Massage
p38

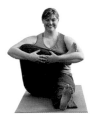

7 Rock the Baby
p40

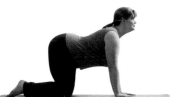

8 Cat and Dog Tilts
p50

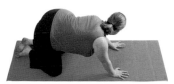

9 Kidney Squeeze
p53

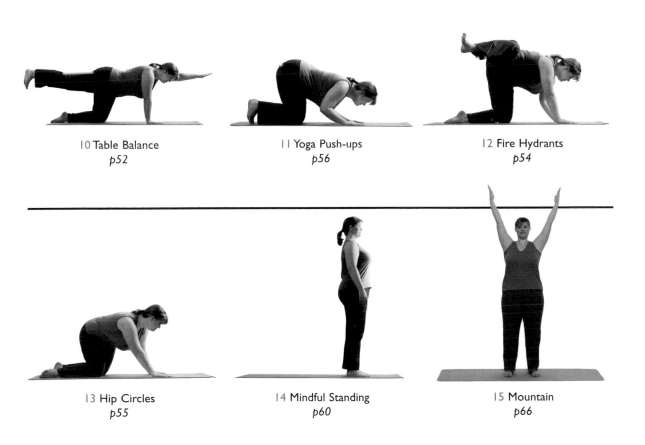

10 Table Balance
p52

11 Yoga Push-ups
p56

12 Fire Hydrants
p54

13 Hip Circles
p55

14 Mindful Standing
p60

15 Mountain
p66

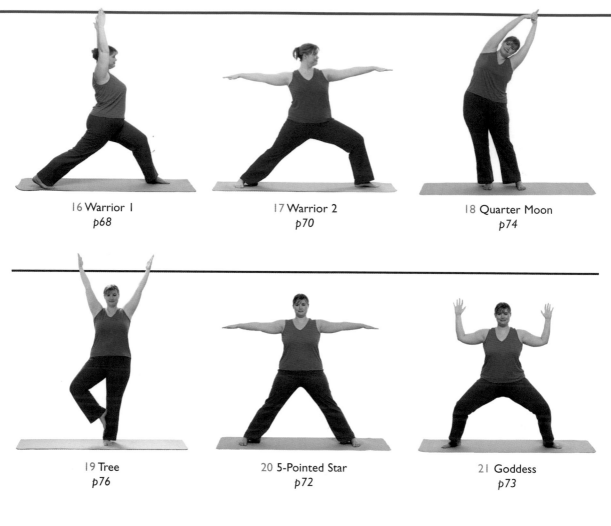

16 Warrior 1
p68

17 Warrior 2
p70

18 Quarter Moon
p74

19 Tree
p76

20 5-Pointed Star
p72

21 Goddess
p73

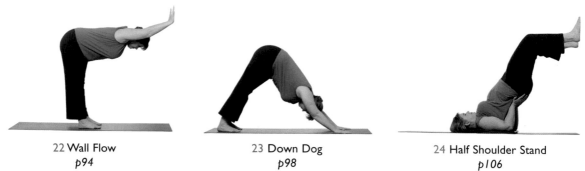

22 Wall Flow
p94

23 Down Dog
p98

24 Half Shoulder Stand
p106

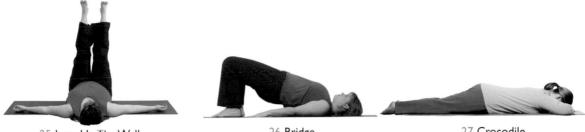

25 Legs Up The Wall
p104

26 Bridge
p112

27 Crocodile
p126

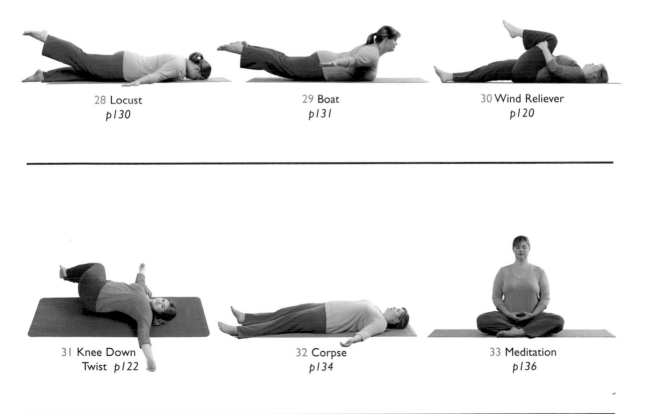

28 Locust
p130

29 Boat
p131

30 Wind Reliever
p120

31 Knee Down
Twist *p122*

32 Corpse
p134

33 Meditation
p136

90-MINUTE PROGRAM

The 90-Minute Program is the workout I use in my personal practice. It will grow with you from months 18 and beyond. This program utilizes all the breathing techniques and postures in the book for a full mind and body experience. In the beginning, use modifications for any poses you have trouble with and then progress to the intensifiers when you are ready for a challenge. If you find a unique sequence that you prefer—go for it! As with the 30-Minute and 60-Minute Programs, start off the 90-Minute Program with centering (see p18) and finish off with several minutes of meditation (see pp136–137).

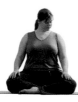
1 Neck Stretches
p32

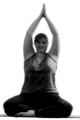
2 Sun Breaths
p34

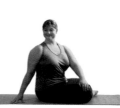
3 Seated Twist
p36

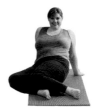
4 Rocking Legs
p37

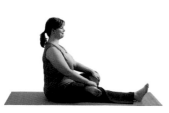
5 Ankle Rolls and Massage
p38

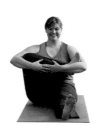
6 Rock the Baby
p40

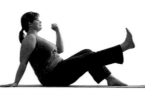
7 Gentle Starfish
p42

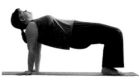
8 Table Top
p46

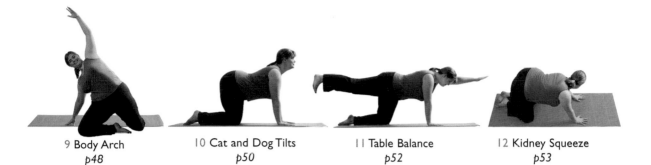

9 Body Arch
p48

10 Cat and Dog Tilts
p50

11 Table Balance
p52

12 Kidney Squeeze
p53

13 Fire Hydrants
p54

14 Hip Circles
p55

15 Yoga Push-ups
p56

16 Child's Pose
p58

17 Underarm Stretch
p59

18 Mindful Standing
p60

19 Mountain
p66

20 Warrior 1
p68

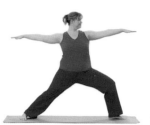

21 Warrior 2
p70

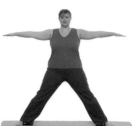

22 5-Pointed Star
p72

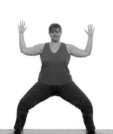

23 Goddess
p73

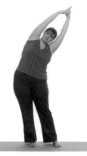

24 Quarter Moon
p74

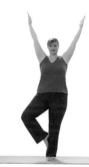

25 Tree
p76

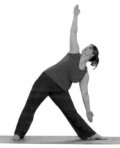

26 Triangle
p78

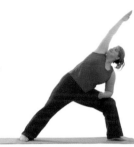

27 Extended Triangle
p80

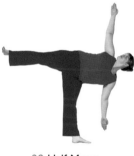

28 Half Moon
p82

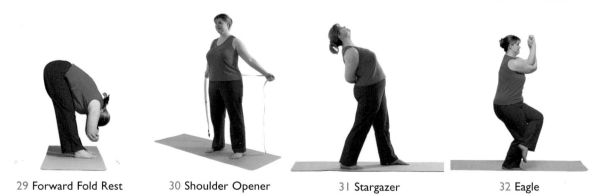

29 Forward Fold Rest
p84

30 Shoulder Opener
p85

31 Stargazer
p86

32 Eagle
p88

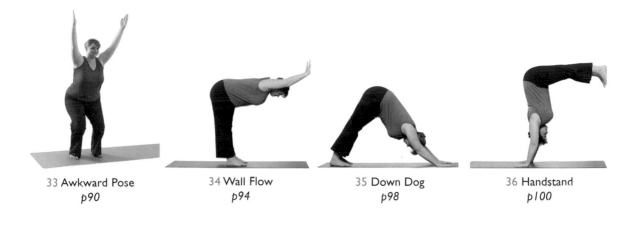

33 Awkward Pose
p90

34 Wall Flow
p94

35 Down Dog
p98

36 Handstand
p100

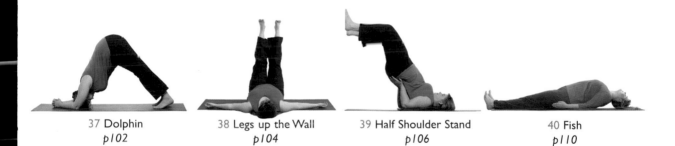

37 Dolphin
p102

38 Legs up the Wall
p104

39 Half Shoulder Stand
p106

40 Fish
p110

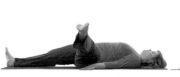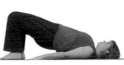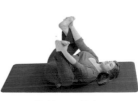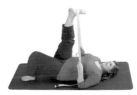

41 Reclining Leg Circles
p111

42 Bridge
p112

43 Happy Baby
p114

44 Reclining Leg Stretch
p116

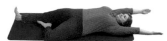

45 Reclining Tree
p118

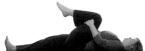

46 Wind Reliever
p120

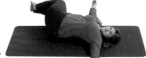

47 Knee Down
Twist *p122*

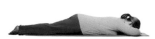

48 Crocodile
p126

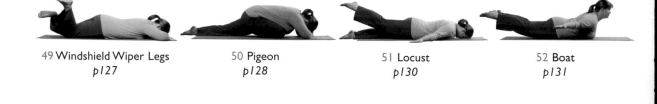

49 Windshield Wiper Legs
p127

50 Pigeon
p128

51 Locust
p130

52 Boat
p131

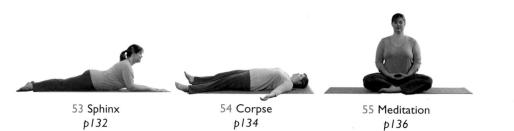

53 Sphinx
p132

54 Corpse
p134

55 Meditation
p136

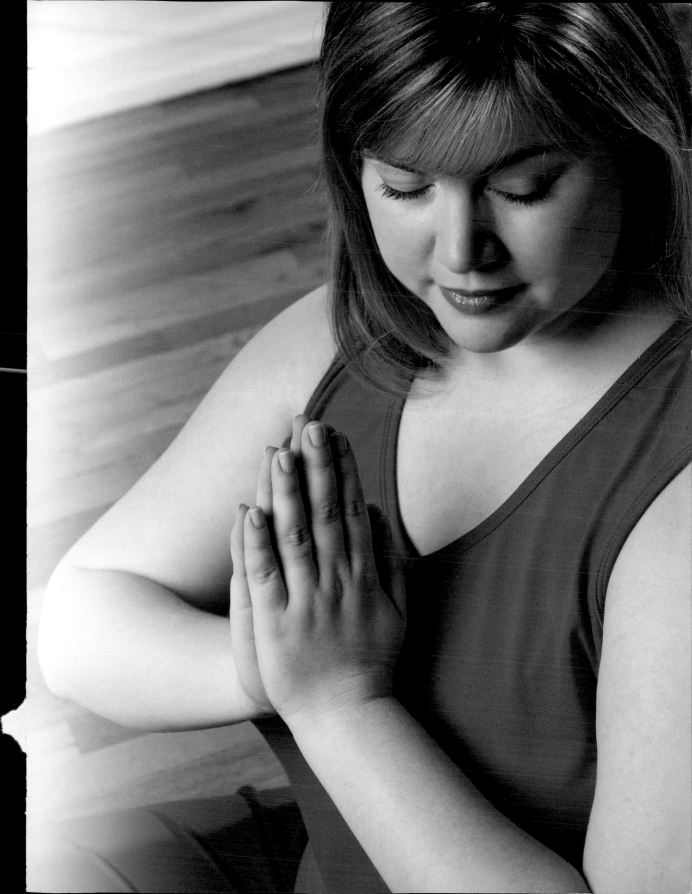

RESOURCES

Look out for yoga classes at your local gym or yoga studio, or, if you're in Manhattan, swing by my class. You can also check out my website (www.megayoga.com) to get updates on class times and locations. For tips on how to find the right class for you, regardless of where you live, take a look at Finding a Teacher. I also share some of my favorite books, instructional DVDs, music, sources for plus-size workout wear, and contact information for yoga retreats.

FINDING A TEACHER

When you are ready to head out into your community and take a yoga class, see if you can audit first or take a free or low-cost trial class. Finding a place where you feel welcomed is a challenge for the plus-size practitioner who oftentimes feels like she stands out like a sore thumb! Look for classes "for round bodies" or "plus-size." Classes for beginner level are another great place to start. If you can find a Kripalu- or Iyengar-trained instructor I highly recommend them.

BOOKS

Yoga Philosophy

Will Yoga and Meditation Really Change My Life?
edited by Stephen Cope, A Kripalu
Book, Storey Publishing, 2003
25 Yoga and meditation teachers explain how the contemplative path has changed their lives. Very revealing and intimate writing.

Silence by Christina Feldman, Roadwell Press, 2003
A gorgeous picture and essay book on silence.

Meditations from the Mat
by Rolf Gates and Katrina Kenison,
Anchor Books, 2002
365 daily meditations to inspire and illuminate your practice time. I often read directly from the entry of the day during the centering of my yoga classes here in New York City.

Loving Kindness: The Revolutionary Art of Happiness
by Sharon Salzberg, Shambhala
Publications, Inc., 2002
In your Megayoga™ practice you will see that I constantly ask you to lift or lighten your heart. Learning Loving Kindness helps make this possible through the wisdom of Buddhist teachings.

Living Your Yoga: Finding the Spiritual in Everyday Life
by Judith Lasater, Ph.D., P.T.,
Rodmell Press, 2000
The most beginner-friendly, easy-to-read explanation of yoga yamas and niyamas (do's and don'ts). My copy is well-worn and well-loved. The yamas and niyamas are a blueprint for better living that yogis practice daily. Have a moral dilemma? Read this book.

Practice

Yoga Body, Buddha Mind by Cyndi Lee,
Riverhead Books, 2004
Cyndi Lee, the founder of Om Yoga Center in New York City is a very lucid, compassionate teacher. This manual of yoga and meditation includes photography of my friend, Catherine Lippincott, a plus-size yogini who masterfully demonstrates the postures.

The Woman's Book of Yoga and Health
by Linda Sparrowe with yoga sequences by
Patricia Walden, Shambhala Publications, 2002
Posture sequences designed for easing PMS, pregnancy, menopause, and post-menopause along with others for women's health and well-being.

Yoga for Women by Shakta Kaur
Khalsa, DK Publishing, 2002

Kundalini Yoga instructor Shakta Kaur Khalsa has produced a beautiful full-color yoga book for all aspects of women's health. I like the little meditations, beauty tips, and students' stories sprinkled throughout.

Alignment and Anatomy

Anatomy of Hatha Yoga by H. David Coulter, Body and Breath, Inc., 2001

The most comprehensive anatomical resource around relating the mechanics of the body to yoga poses. Wondering where your adrenals are? Puzzled about the effects of twists on digestion? It's all in here. Very dense and technical—fascinating.

Yoga Mind, Body, and Spirit by Donna Farhi, An Owl Book, Henry Holt and Company, 2000

Great illustrated asana (posture) book that goes into detail about the effects of the postures on the systems of the body. One of the best explanations of the principles of movement and general alignment.

Light on Yoga by B.K.S. Iyengar, Schocken Books, 1966, 1968, 1976

B.K.S. Iyengar elucidated yoga for students of the West back in the sixties. His original yoga manual on postures, breathing, meditation, and philosophy is the text that thrilled and beckoned me down the path of yoga.

Inspirational Memoir

Pilgrim of Love: The Life and Teachings of Swami Kripalu edited by Atma Jo Ann Levitt, Monkfish Book Publishing Company, 2004

The life story of Bapuji, the yogic sage and namesake of Kripalu Yoga. A great Kundalini yoga master, devoted teacher, and above all pilgrim of God who inspired thousands of Kripalu teachers and students. Swami Kripalu survived a suicide attempt, lived as a family man, found his guru, and became a swami carrying a begging bowl and wearing a loin cloth—all this before the age of 33!

Finding My Balance by Mariel Hemingway, Simon and Schuster, 2003

The granddaughter of Ernest Hemingway writes about her struggles with family alcoholism, suicides, mental illness, and her own eating disorder. Yoga practice helped put her on the path to sobriety and nonviolence. A must-read for all of us who struggle or have struggled with loving ourselves.

Yoga and the Quest for the True Self by Stephen Cope, Bantam Books, 1999

Stephen Cope is a psychotherapist and Kripalu teacher who writes here about his own spiritual growth as a yogi living and working at Kripalu Center. He dances from the personal to the universal, explaining how the mind and body changes, struggles, and suffers on the journey to awakening.

Plan B: Further Thoughts on Faith by Anne Lamott, Riverhead Books, 2005

An irreverent, hilarious collection of essays from author and single mom Anne Lamott, wrestling with living as a Christian while thinking decidedly un-Christian thoughts.

Just for Fun

Self-Nurture by Alice D. Domar, Penguin Books, 2000

Good book of suggestions for taking care of your needs, from basic time management skills to treats for yourself. Helps show you how to be compassionate with yourself. Good chapter on relaxing meditations.

Life's Little Emergencies by Emme Aronson

Emme, the world's first plus-size supermodel, has written a cute book on fashion, beauty, health, and lifestyle. A fun read by a true role model and trailblazer in the plus-size community. Check out the section on yoga—Emme practices, too.

INSTRUCTIONAL DVDS

A.M. and P.M. Yoga for Beginners by Gaiam, with Rodney Yee and Patricia Walden, 1999
Two 20-minute yoga sessions led by master teachers. Rodney leads the enlivening A.M. session in Maui on the beach. Patricia leads the reflective P.M. session in the desert. A classic and national best seller.

Yoga Mind and Body with Ali MacGraw, Warner Home Video, 1994
Ali MacGraw and several students practice, led by Erich Schiffman. The music is by Dead Can Dance. Practice next to a wall and use your props (such as a chair) so you can modify the Sun Salute section.

Yoga Just My Size™ with Megan Garcia, A Born Beautiful production, 2004
My DVD for the plus-size practitioner. A basic, brief daily practice session, like the 30-Minute Program in MegaYoga™. Includes an interview with me and a special tips section.

Kripalu Yoga Gentle and *Kripalu Yoga Intermediate* (VHS format)
These two tapes make perfect gifts. Everyone can do the gentle poses—I gave them to my mom and dad before I made my own DVD. Bare-bones aesthetics—just a studio and great teachers.

INSTRUCTIONAL CDS

Pranayama: The Kripalu Approach to Yogic Breathing (Beginner) by Yoganand Michael Carroll, 2000
My instructor's basic instructional on breathing techniques—Dirgha, Ujjayi, Kapalabhati, and Alternate Nostril. Taught me everything I know about breathing.

MUSIC TO INSPIRE YOUR PRACTICE

Here is a peek at the rotating yoga playlist in my Manhattan classes. Most-requested albums are first.

Shamanic Dream and *Shamanic Dream II* by Anugama, Open Sky Music, 2000
www.openskymusic.com
Primordial, nature sounds, great beat.

Music for Sound Healing by Stephen Halpern, Open Channel Sound Company, 1999
www.innerpeacemusic.com
Synthesizer, very gentle.

Drala [self–titled] produced by David Nichtern and Dharma Moon, 2001
Wonderful for contemplation as well as yoga practice.

Om Yoga Mix sequenced by Cyndi Lee, produced by Dharma Moon, 2003
Sequenced for yoga practice.

Music for Yoga and Other Joys by Jai Uttal and Ben Leinbach, Gemini Sun Records, 2003, distributed by Sounds True, Inc.
Especially the last two tracks—blissful.

Sundari, a Jivamukti Yoga Class by Gabrielle Roth, Raven Recording, 1999
Sequenced for a flow-style class, comes with illustrated class sequence. Very energizing.

SOURCES FOR PLUS-SIZE WORKOUT WEAR

Junonia
www.junonia.com
Plus-size catalog company for exercise clothing.

Just My Size
www.jms.com
Good basics. I buy the tank top with shelf bra and spaghetti straps one size too small so it doesn't ride up as I practice.

Danskin
www.danskin.com
Try the Supplex fabric leggings, very soft.

PROPS

Hugger-Mugger Yoga Products
3937 South 500 West
Salt Lake City, Utah 84123
Tel (800) 473-4888
Fax (801) 268-2629
www.huggermugger.com
Yoga mats, blocks, straps, etc.

Manduka
www.manduka.com
Mats and mat bags.

Yoga Props
www.yogaprops.com
Mats, blocks, straps, etc.

YOGA RETREAT CENTERS

Kripalu Center for Yoga and Health
Lenox, Massachusetts
www.kripalu.org
Everything from great yoga classes to massages to vegetarian gourmet food. Kripalu hosts famous teachers in Buddhism, yoga, and all the contemplative arts.

Himalayan Institute
952 Bethany Turnpike
Honesdale, PA 18431
(570) 253-5551
(800) 822-4547
Email: info@HimalayanInstitute.org
Website: www.himalayaninstitute.org
Retreat in rural Pennsylvania.

PERIODICALS

Yoga Journal
www.yogajournal.com
The classic yoga magazine—I've been a subscriber for many years. It's been around since 1975.

INDEX

ACKNOWLEDGMENTS

AUTHOR'S ACKNOWLEDGMENTS

Many hard-working, talented people made MegaYoga™ possible. I would like to thank the staff at DK: Carl Raymond for discovering me; Jennifer Williams, my editor and fellow Smithie, for her encouragement and patience; Tai Blanche and Michelle Baxter for their artful eyes (and for sticking down mats, smoothing wrinkles, and doing a million other jobs); PR Queen Rachel Kempster and the marketing team for their enthusiasm.

From the shoot, I'd like to thank: our host, Hugh Bell; photographic team extraordinaire Kellie Walsh and Rupert Rogers, whose creativity, positive energy, and professionalism supported a great shoot; make-up artist Tamami Mihara; digital editor Christian-Miles StomsVik; photo & lighting assistant Doug Todd; Elissa K. Meyrich of Sew Fast, Sew Easy, for the colorful wardrobe; Hugger-Mugger for donating top-notch props; Nadine Raphael for the cover shot; Dirk Kaufman for the beautiful cover design; my yoga teachers at Kripalu Yoga, Yoganand Michael Carroll and Tarika Diana Damelio—I hope to change others as you changed me with your teachings and wisdom; teachers past J.J. Gormley and Rodney Yee; teachers via the written word, audio, and video Stephen Cope, Judith Lasater, Cyndi Lee, and Eric Schiffman; my guru, Swami Kripalu, to whom I bow; the big hearts, my students, especially Sheryl Simonitis and Letitia Mateo, from whom the meditations and spirit of the book emerged; my substitute teachers, Ann Megyas and Martina Puchta, for their support; my family—Terry, Gina, Emily, Rhys, and Tad for their love; and—the best for last—Rolando, my husband, my best friend and the love of my life. Why not both? Yes.

PUBLISHER'S ACKNOWLEDGMENTS

DK would like to thank Alex Parra and Hugger-Mugger Yoga Products for generously donating props; John Searcy and Christy Lusiak for their editorial assistance; and Nichole Morford for being so helpful at the shoot; Engly Chang and Erin Harney for help with design and preparing repro files; and Tommy Campbell for a great painting job at the photo studio.

PICTURE CREDITS

The publisher would like to thank Megan Garcia for her kind permission to use photographs from her modeling portfolio on pages 6-7.

ABOUT THE AUTHOR

Megan Garcia fell in love with yoga in her first class at Smith College in the early 1990s. She received teacher training at Kripalu Center in Lenox, Massachusetts, in 1999, and started teaching on Manhattan's Upper West Side soon after. She rapidly developed a following in the community of plus-size women who enjoyed the body-friendly modifications and positive spirit of Megan's teachings. In February 2005, Megan came out with her first DVD, *Yoga: Just My Size*™ *with Megan Garcia.* The DVD created a media sensation, receiving national coverage on *The Today Show*, CNN, MSNBC, and in the pages of national magazines. By day, Megan works as a successful plus-size model for such publications as *Figure Magazine* and *Glamour,* and the style guidebook *Figure It Out.* Her prior clients include Lane Bryant and Fashion Bug. Megan is married and lives in West New York with her husband, Rolando, a martial arts instructor and actor. For more information about Megan and her classes, visit www.megayoga.com.